Questions and Answers for Symptoms and Signs in Clinical Medicine

Questions and Answers for Symptoms and Signs in Clinical Medicine

by

J. E. Earis MD, MRCP

Consultant Physician, Fazakerly and Walton Hospitals, Liverpool

and

Colin Ogilvie MD, FRCP

Consultant Physician to the Royal Liverpool Hospital, the Liverpool Regional Cardiothoracic Centre and the King Edward VII Hospital, Midhurst

WRIGHT

Bristol

1987

Published under the Wright imprint by:
IOP Publishing Limited
Techno House, Redcliffe Way, Bristol BS1 6NX

British Library Cataloguing in Publication Data
Ogilvie, C.
Questions and answers for symptoms and signs.
1. Physical diagnosis——Problems, exercises, etc.
I. Title II. Ears, J.E.
616.07′54′076 RC76

ISBN 0 7236 0865 2

Typeset by:
BC Typesetting, 51 School Road, Oldland Common, Bristol BS15 6PJ

Printed in Great Britain by:
Butler & Tanner Ltd., Frome and London

Preface

The multiple choice question is a notorious device for deciding whether a student passes or fails a professional examination. This little book may provide useful practice for such examinations but this is not its main purpose. The questions have been designed to reveal common errors in clinical diagnosis while the answers—on the reverse side of each page—seek to explain the reasons for these errors. For the sake of variety, we have also put questions in the form of 'pair associations', classic clinical histories and pictures of common physical signs.

The book is intended as a companion volume to the new edition of Chamberlain's *Symptoms and Signs in Clinical Medicine* (11th edition). For easy reference, the chapter headings and numbers are the same in the two books.

We are grateful to those of our colleagues who checked the fairness of our questions and the accuracy of our answers. In particular, we wish to thank Drs J. M. Bone, D. W. Chadwick, D. P. Heaf, M. J. Mackie, A. I. Morris and F. J. Nye.

We are also indebted to the publishers, John Wright, for encouraging us to write this book and for all their help in its preparation.

J. E.
C. O.

Contents

The Chapter numbers in brackets refer to the new 11th Edition of 'Symptoms and Signs in Clinical Medicine'

External Manifestations of Disease

(Refer to Chapter 3 in *Symptoms and Signs in Clinical Medicine*, 11th edition, p. 36.)

1. Puffiness around the eyes is a characteristic feature of

a. Myxoedema
b. Cushing's syndrome
c. Acne rosacea
d. Superior vena caval obstruction
e. Allergic reaction to drugs

2. Unilateral exophthalmos is a recognized feature of

a. Glaucoma
b. Orbital tumours
c. Primary hyperthyroidism
d. Thrombosis of the cavernous sinus
e. Retinal vein thrombosis

3. Conjunctivitis sicca is

a. Confirmed by the Schirmer test
b. Always present in Sjögren's syndrome
c. A recognized complication of measles
d. Caused by blocked lacrimal ducts
e. A recognized feature of hay fever

4. Arcus senilis is

a. Due to lipoid material obscuring the periphery of the iris
b. A typical feature of old age
c. A complication of iritis
d. A recognized complication of measles
e. Seen more frequently in Africans than Europeans

5. Angular stomatitis is a recognized complication of

a. Addison's disease
b. Vitamin E deficiency
c. Ill-fitting dentures
d. Oral candidiasis
e. Ariboflavinosis

Answers overleaf

1. (*a, d, e*)
Puffiness of the eyelids is commonly seen in myxoedema, renal disease and as part of an allergic reaction to drugs, foods and insect bites. With superior vena caval obstruction the whole head and neck may be suffused and oedematous. The 'moon face' of Cushing's syndrome and the typical butterfly rash of rosacea are not characteristically associated with oedema of the eyelids.

2. (*b, c, d*)
Unilateral exophthalmos is usually the first sign of an orbital tumour and the marked chemosis and proptosis of cavernous sinus thrombosis is a very dramatic physical sign. Unilateral exophthalmos is also well recognized in primary hyperthyroidism although this usually progresses to the more typical bilateral involvement. Glaucoma is caused by high intra-occular pressure and is not associated with exophthalmos.

3. (*a, b*)
Conjunctivitis sicca (abnormal dryness of the eyes) is due to lacrimal gland disease (e.g. Sjögren's syndrome). The diagnosis is confirmed by placing a small strip of sterile filter paper under the lower eyelid and demonstrating reduced lacrimal secretion (Schirmer's test). Watering (epiphoria) of the eyes is associated with measles, hay fever and blockage of the lacrimal or tear duct.

4. (*a, b, c, e*)
As its name implies arcus senilis most commonly occurs in the elderly. It is due to deposition of lipoid material and is seen in hyperlipidaemia. There is a higher incidence in African than European populations and it is not associated with iritis.

5. (*c, d, e*)
Angular stomatitis, especially when associated with glossitis, may indicate ariboflavinosis. However, the commoner causes of this condition are ill-fitting dentures and oral candidiasis.

6. Which of the following statements about herpes simplex are true?

a. Primary infection usually occurs in utero.
b. It is a recognized feature of respiratory tract infections.
c. The skin lesions are non-infective.
d. Recurrent attacks may be triggered by minor trauma.
e. Encephalitis is usually a trivial illness.

7. Lupus pernio

a. Is caused by *Mycobacterium tuberculosis*.
b. May cause excessive destruction of the nose.
c. In nearly every case is associated with skin ulceration.
d. Is associated with rhinophyma (strawberry nose).
e. Is associated with nasal polyps.

8. Acne rosacea is

a. Associated with high alcohol intake
b. Characterized by butterfly-wing rash
c. Typically accompanied by systemic manifestations
d. An associated cause of keratitis
e. Is commonly seen in adolescents

9. Nasal polyps are associated with

a. Bronchial asthma
b. Polyposis coli
c. Carcinomatous change
d. Massive haemoptysis
e. Children rather than adults

10. Gouty tophi

a. Typically occur on the ears.
b. May discharge urate crystals.
c. Are characteristically associated with symmetrical joint swelling.
d. Usually occur without gouty attacks.
e. May be accompanied by renal impairment.

Answers overleaf

6. (*b, d*)
Herpes simplex (type 1) is a DNA virus usually acquired in childhood, the primary infection presenting as an ulcerative stomatitis. The virus may remain dormant in the trigeminal root ganglion until reactivated (e.g. by a respiratory tract infection or mild trauma) when it produces ulcerative vesicular lesions around the mouth which contain live virus. Herpes encephalitis is a very serious and often fatal infection.

7. (*b*)
Lupus pernio is a sarcoid granulomatous lesion which, like lupus vulgaris (due to *Mycobacterium tuberculosis*), causes extensive destruction of the nose although very rarely results in skin ulceration. Rhinophyma (strawberry nose) is associated with acne rosacea.

8. (*a, b, d*)
Acne rosacea occurs in the blush area (face, neck and upper chest) often producing a butterfly-wing rash on the face. It is not associated with systemic disease, the most serious complication being local involvement of the eyes (keratitis) which can result in visual failure. Although alcohol does not cause rosacea it can aggravate the condition. It is acne vulgaris that is commonly seen in adolescents.

9. (*a*)
Nasal polyps are frequently associated with bronchial asthma in adults but are rare in childhood. They usually present with nasal obstruction and are not complicated by massive epistaxis or carcinomatous changes. There is no association with polyposis coli.

10. (*a, b, e*)
Tophaceous gout is always associated with recurrent acute gouty attacks which are characterized by asymmetrical joint involvement. Tophi are subcutaneous collections of sodium urate crystals which occasionally ulcerate and discharge their contents. They typically occur on the ear lobes, around the affected joints and on bursae and tendons. Renal impairment and calculi are common complications of gout (about 25 per cent of these patients die from renal failure).

11. Salivary gland enlargement is a recognized feature of

a. Typhoid fever
b. Sarcoidosis
c. Sjögren's syndrome
d. Ramsay Hunt syndrome
e. Leukaemias

12. Congenital syphilis is characteristically associated with

a. Increased incidence of hydrocephalus
b. Frontal bossing of the skull
c. Depression of the bridge of the nose
d. Pink fluorescence of the teeth
e. Nerve deafness

13. Which of the following statements about 'lumps' in the neck are true?

a. A goitre can always be felt in the neck.
b. Sarcoid lymph nodes are tender.
c. Bronchial carcinoma very rarely spreads to the cervical nodes.
d. 'Rubbery' enlargement of lymph nodes is characteristic of lymphoma.
e. A thyroid swelling moves upwards on swallowing.

14. Hair loss is a recognized feature of

a. Hypothyroidism
b. Secondary syphilis
c. Cushing's syndrome
d. Chronic hepatic failure
e. Hypoparathyroidism

15. Short stature is characteristic of

a. Eunuchoidism
b. Chronic steroid-dependent childhood asthma
c. Marfan's syndrome
d. Cystic fibrosis
e. Ovarian dysgenesis (Turner's syndrome)

Answers overleaf

11. (*a, b, c, e*)
Inflammation of the salivary glands is most commonly due to mumps but can also be secondary to typhoid fever and other bacterial infections. Enlargement of the salivary glands is occasionally present in sarcoidosis, Sjögren's syndrome, leukaemias and in patients with alcoholic cirrhosis. The Ramsay Hunt syndrome is caused by herpes zoster of the geniculate ganglion.

12. (*b, c, e*)
Congenital syphilis is now very rare. The child often appears normal at birth, later developing various stigmata of the disease. These include bony deformities of the skull, notched teeth (pink fluorescence is caused by congenital porphyria), iritis, keratitis and various neurological abnormalities.

13. (*d, e*)
Cervical lymphadenopathy in adults frequently represents serious underlying disease. The glands are usually painless and if due to carcinoma (most commonly carcinoma of the bronchus) are very hard and irregular. Rubbery nodes are characteristic of sarcoidosis, lymphoma and leukaemias. A goitre moves upwards on swallowing but may be entirely retrosternal in site.

14. (*a, b, d*)
The causes of hair loss (alopecia) include local diseases of the scalp, endocrine disorders (myxoedema, hypopituitarism and Addison's disease), liver disease, syphilis, treatment with drugs (e.g. cytotoxic agents and heparin) and radiotherapy. Cushing's syndrome is associated with an excess of hair.

15. (*b, d, e*)
Eunuchoidism and Marfan's syndrome are both associated with tall thin build. Short stature is seen in extreme form (dwarfism) in achondroplasia and anterior pituitary failure in children. Cystic fibrosis, childhood steroid therapy and Turner's syndrome are further causes of short stature.

16. Obesity may be a factor in the development of

a. Diabetes mellitus
b. Gout
c. Gallstones
d. Fatty liver
e. Uterine prolapse

17. Pigmentation is an associated feature of

a. Hypopituitarism
b. Lead poisoning
c. Intestinal malabsorption
d. Addison's disease
e. Therapeutic irradiation

18. Flushing of the skin is characteristic of

a. The menopause
b. Carcinoid tumours
c. Hypothyroidism
d. Hypercarbia
e. Alcoholism

19. Which of the following statements concerning skin rashes are true?

a. Herpes zoster is associated with infection of the posterior root ganglion.
b. Bullous eruptions are sometimes due to drug overdose.
c. Pustules in acne vulgaris are caused by infection.
d. Nicotinic acid deficiency is associated with a skin rash.
e. *Café-au-lait* spots are a characteristic feature of neurofibromatosis (von Recklinghausen's disease).

20. Erythema nodosum is a recognized complication of

a. Sarcoidosis
b. Treatment with sulphonamide drugs
c. Inflammatory bowel disease
d. Streptococcal infections
e. Tuberculosis

Answers overleaf

16. (*a, c, e*)
Obesity is associated with the development of many diseases but not gout or fatty liver, the latter usually being a manifestation of alcoholic liver disease.

17. (*c, d, e*)
Increased pigmentation is a feature of many conditions. Hypopituitarism, however, usually results in reduced pigmentation, while lead poisoning causes pallor due to anaemia and may also be associated with a blue-black lead line on the gingival margins of the teeth.

18. (*a, b, d, e*)
Flushing, mainly of the head and neck, is commonly seen with emotion and as a menopausal symptom. Carcinoid tumours (usually in the presence of extensive hepatic metastases) cause flushing due to the release of tryptophan metabolites. More generalized flushing occurs in hypercarbia, hyperthyroidism (not hypothyroidism) and alcoholism.

19. (*a, b, d, e*)
The herpes zoster virus which is dormant in the posterior root ganglion following childhood chickenpox may become reactivated producing the typical vesicular rash in the affected dermatone. Bullous eruptions are sometimes seen in barbiturate and occasionally other drug overdoses. Pustules in acne vulgaris are not typically infected, but are caused by sterile inflammatory reaction secondary to inspissated sebum blocking the sebaceous glands. *Café-au-lait* spots are pigmented macules of more than 1 cm in diameter.

20. (All correct)
Erythema nodosum is a vasculitic rash that most commonly affects the shins. It is frequently associated with sarcoidosis but also occurs after streptococcal infections, tuberculosis, the administration of sulphonamide drugs and inflammatory bowel disease. It is always self-limiting.

21. Which of the interpretations of the following physical signs are correct?

a. Heberden's nodes are typical of rheumatoid arthritis.
b. Gangrene of the fingers is typically associated with atheroma.
c. Arachnodactyly is one of the diagnostic features of Turner's syndrome (ovarian dysgenesis).
d. Yellow nail syndrome is associated with pleural effusions.
e. Leukonychia is a recognized feature of chronic liver failure.

22. Which of the following statements concerning the legs are correct?

a. Loss of hair is associated with arterial ischaemia.
b. Purpura is seen more frequently on the arms than the legs.
c. Pes cavus is a common accompaniment of syringomyelia.
d. Sabre tibia is a diagnostic feature of syphilis.
e. Paget's disease is associated with knock-knees.

Answers overleaf

21. (*d, e*)
Heberden's nodes which are found around the terminal interphalangeal joints may be associated with osteoarthritis. Gangrene of the fingers is rarely due to atheromatous occlusion of the larger arteries of the arms, but more often to damage of smaller blood vessels (e.g. arteritis secondary to scleroderma and rheumatoid arthritis). Ergot poisoning is another very rare cause. Arachnodactyly is seen in Marfan's not Turner's syndrome. Yellow nail syndrome is a rare condition associated with lymphoedema frequently accompanied by pleural effusions. Any cause of hypoproteinaemia including liver disease may cause white nails (leukonychia).

22. (*a, c, d*)
Purpura (due to bleeding into the skin) is most commonly seen on pressure areas (e.g. buttocks) and on the lower legs. Paget's disease is associated with bow legs rather than knock-knees. Pes cavus is characteristic of congenital neurological diseases like syringomyelia and hereditary ataxias. Sabre tibia (anterior bowing of the shins) is seen in late congenital syphilis.

Arrange the following associations into their correct pairs:

1.	*A*. Puffiness around the eyes	*a*. Sarcoidosis
	B. Unilateral exophthalmos	*b*. Bronchial asthma
	C. Angular stomatitis	*c*. Hyperthyroidism
	D. Lupus pernio	*d*. Ariboflavinosis
	E. Nasal polyps	*e*. Myxoedema
2.	*A*. Tophi	*a*. Syphilis
	B. Saddle nose	*b*. Sarcoidosis
	C. Butterfly-wing rash	*c*. Rickets
	D. Parotid swelling	*d*. Systemic lupus erythematosus
	E. Frontal bossing of the skull	*e*. Gout
3.	*A*. Hair loss	*a*. Turner's syndrome
	B. Short stature	*b*. Barbiturate overdose
	C. Skin pigmentation	*c*. Tuberculosis
	D. Erythema nodosum	*d*. Hypothyroidism
	E. Bullous eruption	*e*. Addison's disease
4.	*A*. Blue sclerotics	*a*. Hypocalcaemia
	B. Argyll Robertson pupil	*b*. Fragilitas ossium
	C. Conjunctivitis sicca	*c*. Hepatolenticular degeneration
	D. Kayser–Fleischer ring	*d*. Sjögren's syndrome
	E. Cataract	*e*. Syphilis
5.	*A*. Flushing	*a*. Neurofibromatosis
	B. *Café-au-lait* spots	*b*. Hodgkin's disease
	C. Pruritus	*c*. Carcinoid tumour
	D. Telangiectasia	*d*. Herpes zoster
	E. Vesicular rash	*e*. Systemic sclerosis
6.	*A*. White nails	*a*. Marfan's syndrome
	B. Arachnodactyly	*b*. Syphilis
	C. Heberden's nodes	*c*. Bacterial endocarditis
	D. Splinter haemorrhages	*d*. Cirrhosis of the liver
	E. Sabre tibia	*e*. Osteoarthritis

Answers overleaf

1. *A......e*
B......c
C......d
D......a
E......b

2. *A......e*
B......c
C......d
D......b
E......a

3. *A......d*
B......a
C......e
D......c
E......b

4. *A......b*
B......e
C......d
D......c
E......a

5. *A......c*
B......a
C......b
D......e
E......d

6. *A......d*
B......a
C......e
D......c
E......b

7. *A*. Hutchinson's teeth
B. Macroglossia
C. Aphthous ulceration
D. Blue line on gums
E. Gum hypertrophy

a. Amyloidosis
b. Lead poisoning
c. Syphilis
d. Crohn's disease
e. Leukaemias

Answers overleaf

7. *A*......*c*
B......*a*
C......*d*
D......*b*
E......*e*

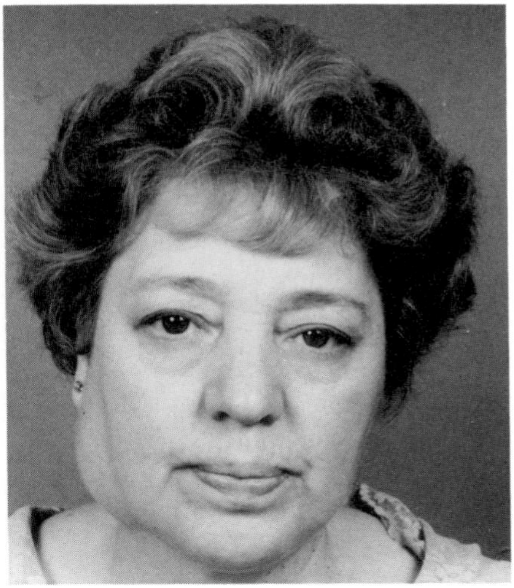

Fig. 3.1
a. What is the likely anatomical site of the abnormality shown?
b. List three possible causes for this appearance.

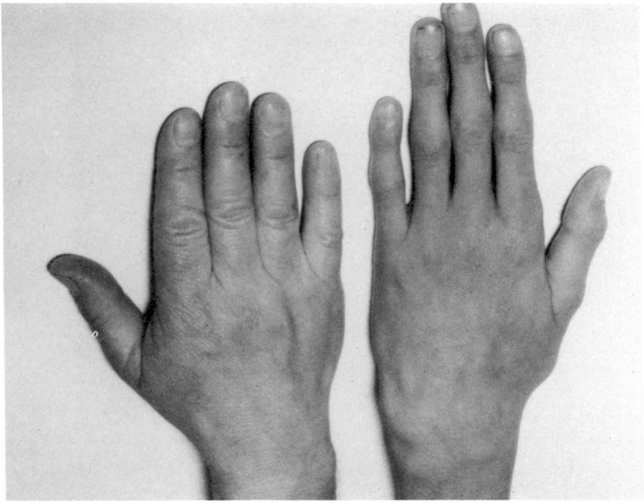

Fig. 3.2
a. What name is given to the appearance of the abnormal hand?
b. Of which syndrome is this a part?

Answers overleaf

Fig. 3.1
a. The right parotid gland
b. Parotid tumour; salivary calculus; systemic causes (mumps, leukaemia, sarcoid, Sjögren's syndrome)

Fig. 3.2
a. Arachnodactyly
b. Marfan's syndrome

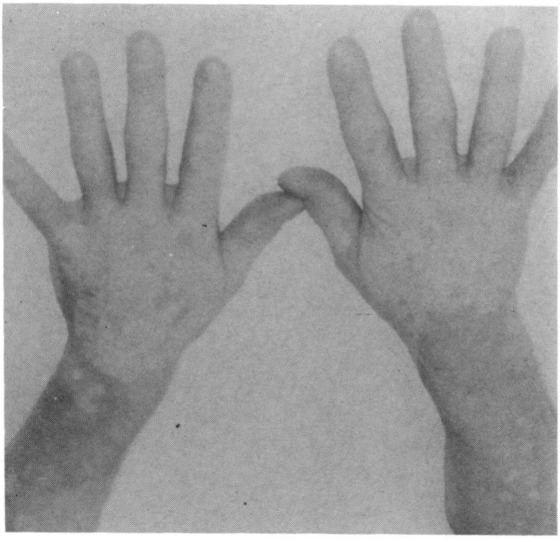

Fig. 3.3
a. What name is given to this skin condition?
b. With which systemic disorders may it be associated?

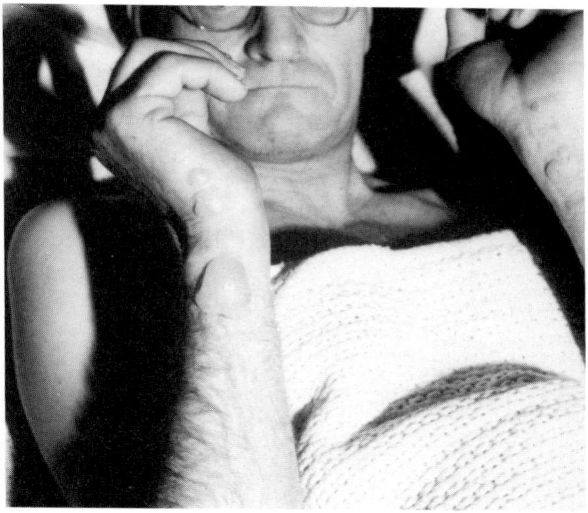

Fig. 3.4
a. How would you describe this type of skin eruption?
b. Give three possible causes.

Answers overleaf

Fig. 3.3
a. Vitiligo
b. Neoplasia or vasculitic conditions

Fig. 3.4
a. Bullous
b. Burns; drug reactions; pemphigus; erysipelas

The Digestive System

(Refer to Chapter 4 in *Symptoms and Signs in Clinical Medicine*, 11th edition, p. 65.)

1. Xerostoma (excessive dryness of the mouth) is a characteristic feature of

a. Parkinsonism
b. Mumps
c. Sjögren's syndrome
d. Stomatitis
e. Sarcoid involvement of the salivary glands

2. Loss of taste

a. Is a feature of a lesion in the 12th cranial nerve.
b. Is a recognized symptom of nasal obstruction.
c. Occurs as an aura in epilepsy.
d. Is a recognized side-effect of certain drugs.
e. Often results in anorexia.

3. Which of the following statements about the teeth and gums are correct?

a. Pink fluorescence is associated with administration of tetracycline in childhood.
b. Gum hypertrophy may result from administration of phenytoin.
c. A blue line in the gums is due to cadmium sulphide.
d. The gums are soft, spongy and bleed easily in vitamin D deficiency.
e. Lung abscess is a recognized complication of oral sepsis.

4. Macroglossia is a recognized feature of

a. Mongolism
b. Amyloidosis
c. Cretinism
d. Syphilis
e. Carcinoma of the tongue

Answers overleaf

1. (*b, c, e*)
Xerostoma is part of Sjögren's syndrome (dry eyes and mouth frequently associated with polyarthritis). Other causes include sarcoidosis and mumps. Parkinsonism and stomatitis cause increased salivation.

2. (*b, d, e*)
The sensation of taste is carried mainly by the 7th and 9th cranial nerves not the 12th (the hypoglossal nerve is the motor nerve to the tongue). Much of what we perceive as 'taste' is in fact smell (1st cranial nerve) and this explains why nasal obstruction is associated with this symptom. Certain drugs (e.g. penicillamine) also affect taste. Temporal lobe epilepsy is occasionally associated with abnormal but not loss of taste.

3. (*b, e*)
As previously mentioned, pink fluorescence of the teeth is associated with congenital porphyria. Tetracycline administered early in life may result in a mottled brownish appearance. Cadmium sulphide may cause a yellow line on the gingival margin, the blue-black line being characteristic of lead poisoning. Gum hypertrophy is an unsightly complication of long-term administration of phenytoin. Spongy haemorrhagic gums are associated with vitamin C deficiency (vitamin D deficiency causes rickets or osteomalacia). Lung abscess in some patients is thought to be caused by inhalation of infected material from the mouth.

4. (*a, b, c*)
Macroglossia is seen in acromegaly, myxoedema, cretinism, mongolism and amyloidosis, but is not a feature of syphilis or carcinoma.

5. Which of the interpretations of the following physical signs concerning the tongue are correct?

a. Depapillated tongue (glossitis) is a feature of severe iron deficiency anaemia.
b. Leucoplakia is of no clinical significance.
c. Ulceration affecting the tip of the tongue is characteristically tuberculous.
d. Aphthous ulceration is usually painless.
e. Geographical tongue is a premalignant condition.

6. Buccal pigmentation is a recognized feature in

a. Cushing's syndrome
b. Normal people
c. Haemochromatosis
d. Peutz–Jegher syndrome (intestinal polyposis)
e. Lead poisoning

7. Stomatitis is a recognized complication of

a. Ill-fitting dentures
b. Treatment with antibiotics
c. Kalar-azar
d. Vitamin B-complex deficiency
e. Leukaemia

8. Dysphagia may result from

a. Aortic aneurysm
b. A goitre
c. Vitamin B_{12} deficiency
d. Systemic lupus erythematosus
e. Bilateral strokes

9. Which of the following statements about oesophageal symptoms are correct?

a. Dysphagia due to tumours is initially more severe when eating solids.
b. With achalasia dysphagia is characteristically variable.
c. Dysphagia is a recognized feature of severe iron deficiency anaemia.
d. Oesophagitis is relieved by stooping and lying flat.
e. Pain from the oesophagus can mimic cardiac pain.

Answers overleaf

5. (*a, c*)
Depapillated tongue may be seen with any severe anaemia. Leucoplakia (hyperkeratosis) may be syphilitic or premalignant, while geographical tongue is relatively common and of no particular clinical significance. Tuberculous ulceration of the tip of the tongue is now very rare, but the small very painful aphthous ulcers are common and sometimes associated with underlying inflammatory bowel disease.

6. (*b, c, d*)
Buccal pigmentation is a classic feature of Addison's but not Cushing's syndrome. It is seen in some normal people (especially Negroes), rarely in haemochromatosis and as discrete patches in the Peutz–Jegher syndrome. Lead poisoning is associated with pallor due to anaemia.

7. (All correct)
These are some of the many recognized causes of stomatitis.

8. (*a, b, e*)
Dysphagia (difficulty in swallowing) has many causes, but these do not include vitamin B_{12} deficiency nor systemic lupus erythematosus. Bilateral strokes are commonly associated with swallowing difficulties due to an upper motor neurone paralysis of the muscles supplied from the medulla or bulb ('pseudobulbar palsy').

9. (*a, b, c, e*)
Dysphagia due to tumours is classically worse when eating solids, although equal difficulty with both solids and liquids together with marked variation in the severity of symptoms is characteristic of achalasia. Iron deficiency may lead to severe symptoms often as part of the Plummer–Vinson syndrome (iron deficiency, dysphagia and oesophageal webs). Oesophagitis is usually made worse by stooping and can mimic cardiac pain (the same segments of the spinal cord receive sensations from both the oesophagus and the heart).

10. Which of the following statements concerning the oesophagus are true?

a. Carcinoma affects the lower one-third in nearly every case.
b. Nocturnal cough is a symptom of oesophageal obstruction.
c. Oesophageal rupture is typically associated with surgical emphysema of the neck.
d. Hiatus hernia is more common in kyphoscoliosis.
e. Achalasia is associated with degeneration of Auerbach's plexus.

11. Which of the following statements relating to abdominal pain are correct?

a. Movement tends to relieve the pain of perforation.
b. Renal colic has a relatively slow onset.
c. Peptic ulcer pain is characteristically exacerbated by vomiting.
d. Shock is a characteristic feature of gallstone colic.
e. Peritoneal inflammation may cause shoulder-tip pain.

12. Vomiting is characteristic of

a. Menière's syndrome
b. Atrophic gastritis
c. Severe hypercalcaemia
d. Severe hyperuricaemia
e. Raised intracranial pressure

13. Haematemesis is a recognized complication of

a. Scleroderma of the stomach
b. Atrophic gastritis
c. Mucosal tear (Mallory–Weiss syndrome)
d. Portal vein thrombosis
e. Administration of aspirin

14. Diarrhoea is a characteristic feature of

a. Zollinger–Ellison syndrome
b. Hirschsprung's disease
c. Heavy metal poisoning
d. Hyperthyroidism
e. Dyschezia

Answers overleaf

10. (*b, c, d, e*)
Although commoner in the lower third, carcinoma may affect any part of the oesophagus. Nocturnal cough due to aspiration of oesophageal contents into the bronchial tree may result in pneumonia and pulmonary fibrosis. Surgical emphysema of the neck can be a very useful clue to the diagnosis of oesophageal rupture. Achalasia is associated with reduction in the myoenteric ganglion cells of the lower oesophagus and a consequent failure of the sphincter to relax.

11. (*e*)
Patients with perforation lie as still as possible because movement increases the pain. Renal colic has a rapid onset and peptic ulcer pain is often relieved and not exacerbated by vomiting. Shock is an uncommon complication of gallstone colic. Because the central part of the diaphragm is supplied by the phrenic nerve (3rd, 4th and 5th cervical segments) inflammation of the overlying peritoneum tends to be referred to the shoulder.

12. (*a, c, e*)
The causes of vomiting do not include atrophic gastritis (which is usually an asymptomatic association of pernicious anaemia) and hyperuricaemia.

13. (*c, d, e*)
By far the commonest cause of haematemesis is a bleeding peptic ulcer. Mucosal tear (Mallory–Weiss syndrome) is the cause in about 10 per cent of cases. Torrential bleeding is seen with oesophageal varices, one cause of which is portal vein thrombosis. Atrophic gastritis and scleroderma of the stomach are not associated with bleeding.

14. (*a, c*)
Diarrhoea is present in the rare Zollinger–Ellison syndrome and is frequently a feature of heavy metal poisoning. Hirschsprung's disease, hypothyroidism and dyschezia all cause constipation and, although faecal incontinence may occur and some liquid stool is sometimes passed (pseudo-diarrhoea), diarrhoea is never the characteristic feature of these conditions.

15. Which of the following statements relating to gallstones are correct?

a. Gallstone colic is continuous rather than intermittent.
b. More than 50 per cent of gallstones are radio-opaque.
c. Gallstone colic may radiate to the right scapula.
d. Pigment stones are associated with hereditary spherocytosis.
e. Gallbladder stones are nearly always clinically silent.

16. Hepatocellular jaundice is

a. Most frequently due to viral hepatitis
b. Commonly associated with elevation of serum alkaline phosphatase
c. Typically associated with urobilinogen in the urine
d. Characteristically associated with marked elevation of the serum liver enzyme concentrations
e. A feature of Weil's disease

17. Severe obstructive jaundice is typically associated with

a. Dark-coloured stools and urine
b. Intolerable itching
c. Bradycardia
d. Marked elevation of the acid phosphatase
e. Absence of urobilinogen from the urine

18. Which of the following statements concerning jaundice are true?

a. Jaundice associated with Gilbert's syndrome is typically symptomless.
b. Dark coloration of the urine on standing is a recognized feature of haemolytic anaemia.
c. Enlargement of the gallbladder in a jaundiced patient is usually due to gallstones.
d. Hepatocellular jaundice is frequently associated with cholestasis.
e. Obstructive jaundice causes malabsorption of fats.

Answers overleaf

15. (*a, c, d, e*)
Gallstone colic only occurs when a stone is passed into the cystic or common bile ducts. It tends to radiate to the scapula and is not strictly colic as it tends to be a continuous pain. Pigment stones contain calcium bilirubinate and are usually associated with chronic haemolysis. Between 10 and 30 per cent of all gallstones are radio-opaque (i.e. contain calcium).

16. (All correct)
The commonest cause of hepatocellular jaundice is viral hepatitis. This type of jaundice is associated with marked abnormality of hepatocellular function with raised serum bilirubin and liver enzymes and reduction in serum albumin (alkaline phosphatase is frequently raised due to coexistent cholestasis).

17. (*b, c, e*)
Obstructive jaundice is associated with pale stools (due to reduced or absent bile flow) and dark urine containing conjugated bilirubin. Bile salts are thought to be the cause of itching and bradycardia. The alkaline not acid phosphatase is elevated (acid phosphatase is derived from the prostate).

18. (*a, b, d, e*)
Gilbert's syndrome (deficiency of glucuronyl transferase) is common and asymptomatic. Urine from patients with haemolytic anaemia becomes discoloured on standing because of the oxidation of urobilinogen. Gallbladder enlargement in a jaundiced patient is very rarely due to gallstones (Courvoisier's law). Cholestasis is associated with fat malabsorption.

19. When inspecting the abdomen:

a. Abdominal distension due to obesity is typically associated with an everted umbilicus.
b. Abdominal striae are a feature of Cushing's syndrome.
c. Caput medusae is a characteristic feature of inferior vena caval obstruction.
d. Peristaltic waves moving from left to right across the abdomen is a recognized feature of pyloric stenosis.
e. Unequal movement of the left and right sides of the abdomen is a recognized feature of unilateral phrenic paralysis.

20. A palpable liver may be caused by

a. Cirrhosis
b. Emphysema
c. Actinomycosis
d. Phrenic paralysis
e. Right-sided heart failure

21. Painful enlargement of the liver is a characteristic feature of

a. Amyloidosis
b. Malaria
c. Viral hepatitis
d. Hepatic abscess
e. Sarcoidosis

22. Palpable enlargement of the gallbladder commonly accompanies

a. Carcinoma of the head of the pancreas
b. Stones in the common bile duct
c. Empyema of the gallbladder
d. Strawberry gallbladder
e. Carcinoma of the gallbladder

Answers overleaf

19. (*b, d, e*)
The umbilicus is inverted in obesity. The commonest cause of striae is previous abdominal distension (e.g. after pregnancy). In Cushing's syndrome the striae are often purple in colour. Caput medusae is associated with portal vein not inferior vena caval occlusion. With inferior vena caval obstruction dilated veins on the side of the abdomen are characteristic. The peristaltic waves in pyloric stenosis move from left to right and in the opposite direction in large bowel obstruction.

20. (*a, b, c, e*)
Right phrenic paralysis causes upward displacement of the liver. All the other conditions listed result in either hepatomegaly or downward displacement of the liver.

21. (*c, d*)
Painful hepatomegaly results from either rapid enlargement (e.g. right cardiac failure or hepatoma) or inflammation (e.g. hepatitis and liver abscess). Hepatomegaly in carcinoma, malaria, amyloidosis and sarcoidosis is frequently painless.

22. (*a, c, e*)
As mentioned in question 18, gallstones do not usually cause a palpable gallbladder and neither does a strawberry gallbladder (cholesterol deposits in the gallbladder wall).

23. Which of the following statements about auscultating the abdomen are true?

a. Bowel sounds are exaggerated in intestinal obstruction.
b. A venous hum is sometimes heard over a normal liver.
c. A systolic murmur over the lower abdomen typically originates from the aorta or iliac arteries.
d. A bruit is sometimes heard over a hypernephroma.
e. Paralytic ileus can be diagnosed if the bowel sounds are not heard after 1 min auscultation.

24. The following are known to infest the gut

a. Taenia saginata
b. Ascaris lumbricoides
c. Enterobius vermicularis
d. Tinea cruris
e. Ankylostoma duodenale

25. Peptic ulcers

a. Occur more frequently in ABO non-secretors.
b. Are more likely to bleed or perforate in patients with blood group A.
c. Are only seen in the stomach and duodenum.
d. Symptoms can be similar to those produced by hookworm disease.
e. Are usually associated with significant hypochlorhydria.

26. Typical features of the malabsorption syndrome include

a. Finger clubbing
b. Pellagroid skin lesions
c. Osteomalacia
d. Tetany
e. Haemorrhage

27. Recognized causes of intestinal malabsorption include

a. Amyloid disease
b. Abnormal intestinal bacterial flora
c. Colonic diverticula
d. Giardia lamblia infestation
e. Lymphoma of the small bowel

Answers overleaf

23. (*a, c, d*)
An abdominal bruit is usually associated with narrowing of the aorta or iliac arteries. However, hypernephroma (carcinoma of the kidney) and hepatoma are other rarer causes. A venous hum is sometimes heard over portosystemic anastomoses but not over a normal liver. Several minutes of auscultation are required before paralytic ileus can be diagnosed with confidence.

24. (*a, b, c, e*)
Tinea cruris (ringworm) is a fungal infection of the skin while all the others are parasitic worms known to infest the gut. *Taenia saginata* is a tape-worm, *Ascaris lumbricoides* a round-worm, *Ankylostoma duodenale* a hook-worm, while the thread-worm (*Enterobius vermicularis*) which most frequently affects children is the only parasitic worm commonly found in this country.

25. (*a, d*)
Peptic ulceration, which is more common in ABO non-secretors, usually occurs in the stomach or duodenum, but more rarely is found in the oesophagus or jejunum and is associated with hyperchlorhydria not hypochlorhydria. Ulcers have a greater tendency to perforate and bleed in patients with blood group O.

26. (All correct)
Malabsorption has very many clinical manifestations. Apart from finger clubbing, all the ones listed in this question are due to nutritional deficiencies.

27. (*a, b, d, e*)
The commonest cause of malabsorption is gluten-sensitive enteropathy. Other less common causes are Crohn's disease, pancreatic insufficiency, small bowel diverticula (the latter by encouraging bacterial overgrowth), amyloid disease, lymphoma and Giardia lamlia infestation.

28. Which of the following statements relating to Crohn's disease are correct?

a. It most frequently affects the ileocaecal region.
b. Fistula formation is characteristic.
c. Mucosal biopsy characteristically shows caseating granulomas.
d. Stricture formation is unusual.
e. Perianal disease is a typical feature.

29. Ulcerative colitis

a. Usually involves the rectum.
b. May cause colonic stricture formation.
c. Is complicated by carcinoma in some long-standing cases.
d. Spares the small bowel.
e. Is occasionally associated with finger clubbing.

30. Carcinoma of the large intestine

a. Has an extremely poor prognosis even when surgically resectable.
b. Is a recognized complication of familial polyposis coli.
c. Most commonly arises in the ascending colon.
d. May present with anaemia.
e. Arising in the sigmoid colon usually presents as an abdominal mass.

31. Irritable colon

a. Is typically associated with a normal barium meal.
b. Is exacerbated by stress.
c. May mimic carcinoma of the colon.
d. Often presents with recurrent abdominal pain.
e. Is sometimes associated with positive faecal occult blood.

Answers overleaf

28. (*a, b, e*)
Although Crohn's disease can affect any part of the gastro-intestinal tract, it is most frequently diagnosed in the ileocaecal region. Strictures are common and anal lesions occur in 50–80 per cent of cases. Biopsy reveals non-caseating granuloma (caseating granuloma being the hallmark of tuberculosis).

29. (All correct)
Unlike Crohn's disease, ulcerative colitis affects the large bowel (most commonly the rectum). Strictures are very rare, but after 10 years of chronic symptoms the development of colonic carcinoma is ten to twenty times that expected from the general population.

30. (*b, d*)
In surgically resectable cases, carcinoma of the large bowel has a relatively good prognosis (overall 5-year survival being approximately 50 per cent). It occurs in the rectum and sigmoid colon in 70 per cent of cases and in these sites an abdominal mass is a very late feature. Unexplained iron deficiency anaemia is a common presentation of bowel carcinoma. Polyposis coli and to a lesser extent ulcerative colitis predispose to the development of bowel carcinoma.

31. (*a, b, c, d*)
The cause of the irritable bowel syndrome is unknown, but it is made worse by stress. The barium enema is always normal and occult bloods are negative. Pain and alteration of bowel habit are common and thus the syndrome can be confused with neoplasm, ulcerative colitis and diverticulitis.

32. Which of the following statements are true of intestinal obstruction?

a. In small bowel obstruction the plain abdominal X-ray shows multiple fluid levels.
b. Faeculent vomiting is a characteristic feature of large bowel obstruction.
c. Auscultation of the bowel sounds is of most diagnostic value in small bowel obstruction.
d. Diarrhoea is a characteristic feature of large bowel obstruction.
e. Succussion splash is a feature of large bowel obstruction.

33. Acute generalized peritonitis can be mimicked by

a. Myocardial infarction
b. Acute porphyria
c. Thyroid crisis
d. Diabetic ketoacidosis
e. Pleurisy

34. Peritoneal fibrosis

a. Is a recognized complication of treatment with any beta-blocking drug.
b. Is a cause of renal failure.
c. Is caused by some treatments of migraine.
d. Is a known complication of carcinoid syndrome.
e. May mimic a peritoneal tumour.

35. Which of the following statements about colonic diverticula are correct?

a. Diverticulosis is characteristically associated with pain.
b. Diverticulitis is best treated with a low-fibre diet.
c. Diverticula are typically diagnosed by sigmoidoscopy.
d. Diverticular disease may mimic colonic carcinoma.
e. Diverticula are much more common in obese patients.

Answers overleaf

32. (*a, c*)
The abdominal X-ray is most dramatic in small bowel obstruction, where multiple fluid levels are seen and there are associated tinkling bowel sounds. In large bowel obstruction vomiting is not common, the major features being colic and absolute constipation. Faeculent vomiting occurs late in small bowel obstruction while succussion splash is associated with pyloric stenosis.

33. (*a, b, d, e*)
The commonest conditions confused with an acute abdomen are myocardial infarction, pleurisy and diabetic ketoacidosis. Acute porphyria and tabes dorsalis are rare sources of confusion. Thyroid crisis usually presents as severe agitation, tachycardia and vomiting.

34. (*b, c, d, e*)
Peritoneal fibrosis is due to chronic peritonitis and may mimic peritoneal tumours. Causes include practolol (but not other beta-blockers) and methysergide. Renal failure sometimes ensues because of ureteric entrapment in the fibrotic tissue.

35. (*d, e*)
Diverticulosis is present in about one-third of people over 60 years of age, is commoner in the obese, is frequently asymptomatic and is diagnosed by barium enema. Diverticular disease which occurs in only a small proportion of those with diverticulosis may mimic carcinoma and this is the indication for sigmoidoscopy. The cause of diverticulosis is thought to be lack of dietary fibre and hence the treatment is a high-fibre diet.

36. Which of the interpretations of the following physical signs concerning liver disease are true?

a. Oesophageal varices only occur when the portal vein is occluded.
b. Gynaecomastia is a recognized feature of liver disease.
c. Flapping tremor is diagnostic of liver disease.
d. Gross nodularity of the liver suggests hepatoma.
e. Splenomegaly in cirrhosis is usually caused by hepatic vein occlusion.

37. Which of the following statements are true of cirrhosis?

a. The commonest cause in Western countries is alcohol.
b. Haemochromatosis causes cirrhosis by deposition of copper in the liver.
c. Alpha-1 antitrypsin deficiency is a cause of juvenile cirrhosis.
d. Convulsions in patients with hepatic failure should be treated with phenobarbitone.
e. Cirrhosis is a recognized sequel of viral hepatitis.

38. Bilirubin

a. Is derived from the breakdown of haemoglobin.
b. When unconjugated is transported in the blood attached to beta-globulins.
c. Is conjugated in the liver with glucuronic acid.
d. Is converted to urobilinogen by gut bacteria.
e. In the unconjugated form is found in the urine of patients suffering from haemolytic jaundice.

39. Typical features of acute pancreatitis include

a. Severe circulatory collapse
b. Hypoglycaemia
c. Periumbilical bruising
d. Intense agonizing upper abdominal pain
e. Hypercalcaemia

Answers overleaf

36. (*b, d*)
Oesophageal varices are the result of portal hypertension of which portal vein thrombosis is one of the many causes. A flapping tremor of the hands is a feature of liver failure, but is not pathognomonic as it is also seen in carbon dioxide retention due to ventilatory failure. Hepatic vein thrombosis is very rare and not the cause of portal hypertension in cirrhosis.

37. (*a, c, e*)
Cirrhosis is the end-result of many pathological processes, the most common being alcohol; viral hepatitis and alpha-1 anti-trypsin deficiency are rarer causes. Haemochromatosis is due to abnormal iron metabolism (copper deposition is associated with Wilson's syndrome). Convulsions in patients with liver failure are best treated with small doses of diazepam, as phenobarbitone is metabolized in the liver and can aggravate encephalopathy.

38. (*a, c, d*)
Bilirubin is derived from haemoglobin. Initially, because it is water insoluble, it is transported attached to plasma albumin and cannot be excreted by the kidneys. Following conjugation in the liver, most is excreted into the bile and subsequently some is converted by bacteria in the gut to urobilinogen and reabsorbed. The increased turnover of bilirubin in haemolytic anaemia results in relatively large amounts of urobilinogen being excreted by the kidneys.

39. (*a, c, d*)
Acute pancreatitis produces agonizing abdominal pain and is frequently associated with circulatory collapse. In severe cases hypo- (not hyper-) calcaemia occurs because of extensive fat necrosis and mild hyperglycaemia is also usual. Periumbilical bruising is a sign of severe haemorrhagic pancreatitis.

40. Which of the following statements about carcinoma of the pancreas are correct?

a. Jaundice is the commonest presenting symptom of tumours in the body of the pancreas.
b. Thrombophlebitis migrans is a well-recognized complication.
c. Pancreatic exocrine insufficiency is an early manifestation of tumours in the body of the pancreas.
d. It is a cause of lymphangitis carcinomatosis of the lung.
e. When jaundice is present the gallbladder is frequently enlarged.

Answers overleaf

40. (*b, d, e*)
Jaundice is a presenting feature of carcinoma of the head (not body) of the pancreas and the gallbladder may be enlarged. Both thrombophlebitis migrans and lymphangitis carcinomatosis are common with this tumour. Pancreatic exocrine insufficiency is not an early manifestation of lesions in the body of the gland.

1. A 64-year-old lady was admitted to hospital with a 5-week history of painless progressive jaundice. Her urine was dark and stools pale.
a. What is the most likely diagnosis?
b. Name two other probable clinical features.
c. Name two abnormal routine investigations.

2. After a bout of drinking a 54-year-old man presented drunk to casualty. He could not give a coherent history but complained of severe chest pain and was found to have surgical emphysema of the neck.
a. What is the probable diagnosis and what was the likely precipitating cause?
b. Name two other likely physical signs.

3. A 42-year-old man complained of long-standing dysphagia which was always worse under emotional stress. He had foul breath, effort dyspnoea and a troublesome nocturnal cough. There was basal shadowing on his chest X-ray.
a. What is the most likely diagnosis?
b. Name two typical features on a barium meal.
c. What is the cause of his dyspnoea and chest X-ray shadowing?

4. A woman of 32 years with a past history of perianal ulceration presents with weight loss, bouts of abdominal pain and diarrhoea. She had a fever and a mass in the right iliac fossa. Sigmoidoscopy was normal.
a. Name the likely diagnosis.
b. List four other features of this condition.

5. A previously fit 68-year-old man complained of weight loss, anorexia and general lassitude. His haemoglobin was 7·5 g/dl. The blood film showed marked microcytosis. Faecal occult bloods were positive.
a. Give the two most likely diagnoses.
b. What investigations would you ask for?

Answers overleaf

1. *a*. Carcinoma of the head of pancreas
b. (i) Weight loss
(ii) Palpable gallbladder
c. (i) Bilirubin in the urine
(ii) High alkaline phosphatase

2. *a*. (i) Ruptured oesophagus
(ii) Forceful vomiting
b. (i) Signs of left basal effusion
(ii) Signs of shock

3. *a*. Achalasia of the cardia
b. (i) Dilatation of the oesophagus
(ii) 'Beak-like' appearance of the lower end of the oesophagus
(iii) Tertiary contractions
c. Regurgitation and aspiration particularly at night

4. *a*. Crohn's disease.
b. (i) Mouth ulceration
(ii) Malabsorption syndrome
(iii) Fistula formation
(iv) Intestinal obstruction

5. *a*. (i) Carcinoma of the stomach
(ii) Carcinoma of the bowel
b. (i) Gastroscopy
(ii) Barium meal
(iii) Sigmoidoscopy
(iv) Barium enema
(v) Colonoscopy

6. A 32-year-old man for many years had passed three or four motions per day. He looked undernourished, was pale, had finger clubbing and mild abdominal distension. Sigmoidoscopy and rectal biopsy were normal.

a. What is the probable diagnosis?
b. Name three known causes.
c. Give four other typical clinical features.

Answers overleaf

6. *a*. Intestinal malabsorption

b. (i) Gluten enteropathy

(ii) Abnormal bacterial flora

(iii) Chronic pancreatic disease

(iv) After gastrectomy or small bowel surgery

c. (i) Pale bulky stools

(ii) Bone pains

(iii) Peripheral neuropathy

(iv) Peripheral oedema

(v) Pellagroid skin lesions and mouth ulcers

Arrange the following associations into their correct pairs:

1. *A*. Xerostoma
B. Loss of taste
C. Gum hypertrophy
D. Pink fluorescence of the teeth
E. Brownish discoloration of the teeth

a. Porphyria
b. Sjögren's syndrome
c. Administration of tetracycline
d. Administration of phenytoin
e. Ninth cranial nerve lesion

2. *A*. Macroglossia
B. Ulcer on tip of tongue
C. Increased salivation
D. Leucoplakia
E. Buccal pigmentation

a. Parkinson's disease
b. Syphilis
c. Tuberculosis
d. Amyloidosis
e. Peutz–Jegher syndrome

3. *A*. Stomatitis
B. Aphthous ulcers
C. Nocturnal cough
D. Surgical emphysema
E. Hiatus hernia

a. Ulcerative colitis
b. Ariboflavinosis
c. Kyphoscoliosis
d. Achalasia
e. Oesophageal rupture

4. *A*. Shoulder-tip pain
B. Regurgitation
C. Haematemasis
D. Vomiting without nausea
E. Rigors

a. Urinary tract infection
b. Duodenal ulcer
c. Cerebral tumour
d. Oesophageal diverticulum
e. Peritonitis

5. *A*. Steatorrhoea
B. Constipation
C. Pigment gallstones
D. Severe pruritus
E. 'Rice-water' stools

a. Hypothyroidism
b. Cholera
c. Polycythaemia vera
d. Spherocytosis
e. Cystic fibrosis

6. *A*. Palpable gallbladder
B. Excess urobilinogen
C. Cholecystitis
D. Abdominal striae
E. Caput medusae

a. Gallbladder stones
b. Haemolytic anaemia
c. Cushing's syndrome
d. Portal vein thrombosis
e. Carcinoma of the pancreas

Answers overleaf

1. *A......b*
B......e
C......d
D......a
E......c

2. *A......d*
B......c
C......a
D......b
E......e

3. *A......b*
B......a
C......d
D......e
E......c

4. *A......e*
B......d
C......b
D......c
E......a

5. *A......e*
B......a
C......d
D......c
E......b

6. *A......e*
B......b
C......a
D......c
E......d

7. *A*. Painless hepatomegaly
B. Painful hepatomegaly
C. Abdominal bruit
D. Shifting dullness
E. Dysphagia

a. Viral hepatitis
b. Sarcoidosis
c. Achalasia
d. Hypernephroma
e. Ascites

8. *A*. Bowel carcinoma
B. Murphy's sign
C. Megaloblastic anaemia
D. Succussion splash
E. White nails

a. Cholecystitis
b. Cirrhosis of the liver
c. Pyloric stenosis
d. Polyposis coli
e. Crohn's disease

9. *A*. Retroperitoneal fibrosis
B. Cirrhosis of liver
C. Periumbilical bruising
D. Malabsorption
E. Ulcerative colitis

a. Pancreatitis
b. Giardia lamblia infestation
c. Carcinoma of the bowel
d. Alpha-1 antitrypsin deficiency
e. Methysergide side-effect

10. *A*. Thrombophlebitis migrans
B. Flapping tremor
C. Chronic sputum production
D. Hypoglycaemia
E. Hypochlorhydria

a. Pernicious anaemia
b. Fibrocystic disease of the pancreas
c. Carcinomatosis
d. Pancreatic islet cell tumour
e. Liver failure

Answers overleaf

7. *A......b*
B......a
C......d
D......e
E......c

8. *A......d*
B......a
C......e
D......c
E......b

9. *A......e*
B......d
C......a
D......b
E......c

10. *A......c*
B......e
C......b
D......d
E......a

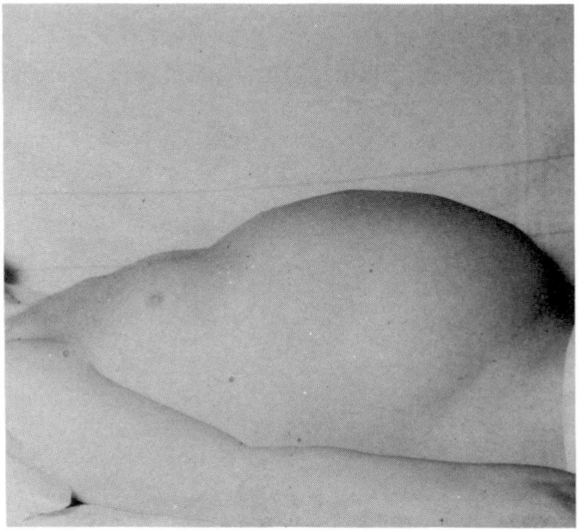

Fig. 4.1
a. What is the most likely cause of this appearance?
b. Give three physical signs which might be found in the abdomen.

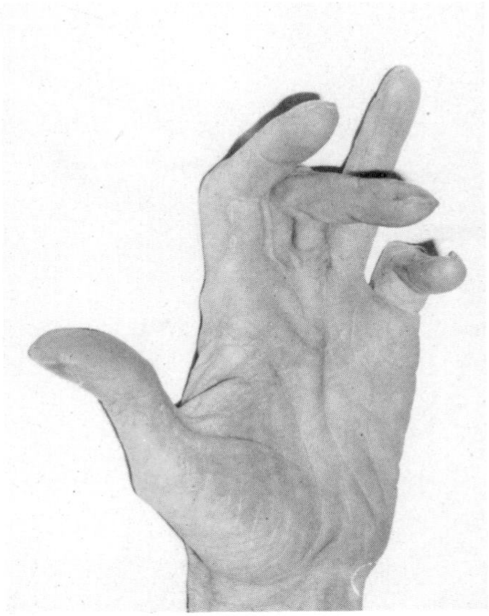

Fig. 4.2
a. Who first described this abnormality?
b. When bilateral, with what abdominal disorder may it be associated?

Answers overleaf

Fig. 4.1
a. Ascites
b. Everted umbilicus; shifting dullness; fluid thrill; neoplastic masses; hepatosplenomegaly

Fig. 4.2
a. Dupuytren (a nineteenth-century French surgeon)
b. Alcoholic hepatic cirrhosis

The Renal and Genital Systems

(Refer to Chapter 5 in *Symptoms and Signs in Clinical Medicine*, 11th edition, p. 131.)

1. Frequency (without increase in the amount of urine) is associated with

a. Bladder tumours
b. Diabetes insipidus
c. Emotional disturbance
d. Acute cortical necrosis
e. Pelvic tumours

2. Retention of urine is a recognized feature of

a. Coma
b. Antidepressant drugs
c. Tabes dorsalis
d. Ureteric calculi
e. Bladder neck obstruction

3. Enuresis is

a. Usually associated with psychological factors
b. Always abnormal after the age of 5 years
c. Best treated with nocturnal fluid restriction
d. Sometimes associated with vesico-ureteric reflux
e. Often associated with frequency during the day

4. The following are causes of incontinence

a. Cerebrovascular disease
b. Multiple sclerosis
c. Traumatic paraplegia
d. Prostatism
e. Prolapsed uterus

5. Polyuria is a characteristic feature of

a. Inappropriate secretion of antidiuretic hormone
b. Diabetes mellitus
c. Nephrogenic diabetes insipidus
d. Chronic renal failure
e. Neurohypophysial diabetes insipidus

Answers overleaf

1. (*a, c, e*)
The causes of passing frequent small amounts of urine during the day and night include infection, bladder tumours, calculi, trauma and reduction in bladder size due to irradiation, pelvic tumours or tuberculosis. Frequency may also result from emotional disturbance but in this case is never associated with nocturia. Acute cortical necrosis results in reduced and diabetes insipidus in increased urine output.

2. (*a, b, c, e*)
Retention of urine occurs in mechanical bladder neck obstruction (e.g. prostatic enlargement and bladder but not ureteric calculi) and may be precipitated by certain drugs with anticholinergic properties (e.g. antidepressants). Neurological causes include tabes dorsalis and other spinal cord lesions.

3. (*a, d, e*)
Enuresis seldom has an organic basis although it is sometimes associated with vesico-ureteric reflux. Frequency during the day is also commonly observed. Ninety per cent of children are dry by the age of 6 years.

4. (All correct)
Incontinence is commonly associated with confusional states either acute or chronic (dementia). Other neurological causes include multiple sclerosis and traumatic spinal cord lesions. Prostatism and prolapsed uterus usually cause less severe types of incontinence, sometimes only occurring after coughing or sneezing.

5. (*b, c, d, e*)
Polyuria is caused by diuresis secondary to high-fluid intake, drugs or the osmotic effect of a high blood sugar in uncontrolled diabetes mellitus. Polyuria also occurs when water resorption in the kidney is impaired, from either chronic renal failure or impaired secretion (or sensitivity to) antidiuretic hormone, as in diabetes insipidus. Inappropriate secretion of antidiuretic hormone is a cause of reduced urine output.

6. Oliguria (less than 500 ml of urine daily) is a recognized complication of

a. Severe hypotension
b. Acute glomerulonephritis
c. Hypercalcaemia
d. Retroperitoneal fibrosis
e. Dissecting aneurysm of the abdominal aorta

7. Renal colic

a. Typically radiates to the hypochondrium.
b. Is commonly associated with vomiting.
c. Is only caused by renal calculi.
d. Is characteristically relieved by lying still.
e. Is a very severe intermittent pain.

8. Which of the following statements about oedema due to renal disease are correct?

a. In acute glomerulonephritis it is typically seen in the face.
b. It is characteristically mild in nephrotic syndrome.
c. It typically occurs when the creatinine clearance is reduced to 80 ml/min.
d. It occurs when the serum albumin is below 25 g/l.
e. It is characteristically non-pitting in chronic glomerular nephritis.

9. Hypertension in renal disease

a. Is usually associated with potassium retention.
b. Is a characteristic feature of acute glomerulonephritis.
c. Is associated with cardiac failure.
d. May result in convulsions.
e. Is associated with papilloedema.

10. Recognized symptoms of renal failure are

a. Thirst
b. Pericardial pain
c. Nausea
d. Kussmaul's breathing
e. Impotence

Answers overleaf

6. (*a, b, d, e*)
Oliguria (passing less than 500 ml of urine a day) occurs with reduced renal perfusion secondary to hypotension or renal artery occlusion, various kidney diseases (e.g. glomerulonephritis) and obstruction of the urinary tract (e.g. retroperitoneal fibrosis). Hypercalcaemia usually causes polyuria.

7. (*b, e*)
Renal colic occurs with acute ureteric obstruction (usually but not exclusively by calculi). It is a severe intermittent pain, often associated with vomiting and, unlike peritonitis, the patient tries to gain relief by moving.

8. (*a, d*)
Pitting oedema is associated with many cases of chronic renal failure (usually when the creatinine clearance is below 5 ml/min). A very low serum albumin and gross oedema are typical of the nephrotic syndrome. In acute glomerulonephritis facial oedema is very common.

9. (*b, c, d, e*)
The hypertension seen in renal disease is nearly always associated with sodium and water retention. It is often very severe in acute glomerulonephritis and can result in heart failure, convulsions and papilloedema.

10. (All correct)
Renal failure affects all body systems and so it is associated with multiple symptoms. Pericardial pain results from uraemic pericarditis, while Kussmaul's breathing is due to hyperventilation associated with the metabolic acidosis of renal failure.

11. The following are typical skeletal complications of renal failure

a. Bone pain
b. Osteomyelitis
c. Subperiosteal resorption of the terminal phalanges
d. Osteomalacia
e. Osteogenesis imperfecta

12. General features of renal failure include

a. Malar flush
b. Muscle twitching
c. Hypoventilation
d. Brownish skin pigmentation
e. Ecchymoses

13. A palpable kidney

a. Invariably signifies an abnormal organ.
b. Moves upwards on inspiration.
c. On the left characteristically causes a dull percussion note on the abdominal wall.
d. Is a typical feature of chronic glomerulonephritis.
e. When due to a hypernephroma is usually cystic.

14. Which of the following statements about the genital tract are correct?

a. Posterior scrotal sinuses strongly suggests genito-urinary tuberculosis.
b. Renal failure is a recognized presentation of carcinoma of the cervix.
c. Genital tuberculosis in the female is almost always associated with urinary tuberculosis.
d. Pruritus vulvae is an early symptom of diabetes insipidus.
e. Testicular tumours are typically painless.

Answers overleaf

11. (*a, c, d*)
Chronic renal insufficiency is associated with abnormal bone metabolism resulting from a mixture of osteomalacia, osteoporosis and secondary hypoparathyroidism. The result may be bone pain or pathological fractures. (Subperiosteal bone resorption of the terminal phalanges is sometimes seen on X-ray.) Osteomyelitis is very uncommon.

12. (*b, d, e*)
General features of a patient with renal failure include pallor, ecchymoses, oedema, brownish skin pigmentation, hyperventilation (Kussmaul's breathing), drowsiness and muscle twitching.

13. (All incorrect)
Normal kidneys may occasionally be palpable particularly on the right. A palpable kidney (which is hard and not cystic when due to a hypernephroma) moves down with respiration, and on the left it can frequently be distinguished from splenomegaly by overlying colonic resonance. The kidneys in chronic glomerulonephritis are typically small.

14. (*a, b, e*)
Posterior tethering of the scrotal skin with sinus formation is pathognomonic of a tuberculous lesion. Unlike males, genital tuberculosis in women is not usually associated with renal involvement. Carcinoma of the cervix produces renal failure by obstructing the ureters. Carcinoma of the testes is typically painless. Pruritus vulvae is associated with diabetes mellitus, not insipidus.

15. When inspecting urine

a. A smoky colour signifies infection.
b. A red colour which fades on standing is characteristic of porphyria.
c. Dark urine is associated with diabetes insipidus.
d. Pink urine occurs in some people after eating beetroot.
e. Turbidity on standing in most cases is due to urates or phosphates.

16. Which of the following statements about urine are correct?

a. Normal specific gravity is typically between 1·015 to 1·025.
b. Urine typically becomes acid after a meal.
c. A fishy smell is associated with the ingestion of shell fish.
d. Glucose is tested by using Ehrlich reagent.
e. Test for ketones is based on colour reaction with nitroprusside.

17. Which of the following statements about proteinuria is correct?

a. In nephrotic syndrome proteinuria typically exceeds 5 g/per 24 h.
b. Orthostatic proteinuria is most marked first thing in the morning.
c. Proteinuria occurs with urinary tract infections.
d. Bence–Jones protein is found in diabetic nephropathy.
e. Normal urine contains up to 1 g of protein per day.

18. Blood in the urine

a. Even in microscopic quantities does not occur in normal people.
b. When associated with dysuria suggests blood is from the kidney.
c. Is tested by the reaction with orthotolidine.
d. Which precedes the urine stream is characteristic of bleeding from the bladder.
e. Is a recognized complication of cystic kidneys.

Answers overleaf

15. (*d, e*)
Smoky urine is associated with blood. Drugs and some foods (e.g. phenolphthalein and beetroot) and porphyria are associated with red coloration; in the case of porphyria the colour darkens on standing. With diabetes insipidus the urine is dilute and pale. On standing, normal urine may become turbid due to the precipitation of phosphates and urates.

16. (*a, e*)
Wide variations in urine specific gravity are normal but typically it is between 1·015 and 1·025. Urine usually becomes alkaline after meals, the so-called alkaline tide. A fishy smell is associated with infection and Ehrlich reagent tests urobilinogen not glucose.

17. (*a, c*)
Normal urine does not contain more than 200 mg of protein daily. Orthostatic proteinuria is thought to be benign and occurs in the upright posture and thus is not present during the night. In the nephrotic syndrome protein loss exceeds 5 g per day; however, in general the extent of renal damage cannot be predicted by the degree of proteinuria. Bence Jones protein is a feature of multiple myeloma.

18. (*c, e*)
On microscopy very small quantities of red cells are seen in normal urine, but this is not enough to produce a positive reaction with orthotolidine. In contrast to the urethra, bleeding from the bladder tends to be at the end of micturition. Bleeding from the kidney is usually painless and can be caused by many renal diseases including polycystic kidneys.

19. The following are recognized causes of pneumaturia

a. *E. coli* urinary tract infections
b. Vesicocolonic fistulae
c. Pneumoperitoneum
d. Pneumocystis coli
e. Renal tuberculosis

20. Casts

a. Are formed by protein precipitating in the tubules.
b. Leucocyte casts are pathognomonic of glomerulonephritis.
c. Red cell casts are a recognized feature of pyelonephritis.
d. Hyaline casts are found in any cause of proteinuria.
e. Red cell casts are best demonstrated after the urine has been standing for several hours.

21. The following crystals may be found in urine:

a. Uric acid
b. Magnesium sulphate
c. Cystine
d. Calcium oxalate
e. Oxalic acid

22. The following are recognized causes of chronic renal failure:

a. Polycystic kidneys
b. Diabetes mellitus
c. Chronic prostatic urethral obstruction
d. Chronic phenacetin medication
e. Pyelonephritis

23. Acute glomerulonephritis is associated with

a. Smoky-coloured urine
b. Hypertension
c. Pulmonary oedema
d. Puffiness of the face
e. Staphylococcal skin infections

Answers overleaf

19. (*b*)
Pneumaturia always suggests a communication between the bladder and the gut. Occasionally it can also occur with urinary infection due to gas-forming organisms, these do not include *E. coli*.

20. (*a, d*)
Casts are formed by protein precipitating in the renal tubules. Hyaline casts can be present in any cause of proteinuria, while red cell casts (the red cells escaping from damaged glomeruli) are pathognomonic of glomerulonephritis and degenerate rapidly if the urine is allowed to stand. Leucocyte casts are typical of pyelonephritis.

21. (*a, c, d*)
Many different crystals may be present in urine including uric acid, calcium oxalate and cystine in patients with cystinuria. Oxalic acid and magnesium sulphate are not seen in urine.

22. (All correct)
Chronic renal failure is the end-result of many different diseases including all those listed. It is particularly important to exclude urinary obstruction as this can usually be treated.

23. (*a, b, c, d*)
Symptoms due to acute glomerulonephritis (inflammation of glomeruli) include blood in the urine (producing a smoky discoloration) and hypertension due mainly to salt and water retention and oedema. Post-streptococcal (not staphylococcal) glomerulonephritis is now becoming increasingly rare.

24. Recurrent haematuria is a feature of

a. Berger's syndrome
b. Prostatic carcinoma
c. Cystic kidneys
d. Renal carcinoma
e. Duplex kidney

25. Diffuse crescentic glomerulonephritis due to Goodpasture's syndrome

a. Runs a relatively benign cause.
b. May be associated with basement membrane antibodies.
c. Is associated with erythema nodosum.
d. Is usually preceded by a sore throat.
e. In some cases is associated with haemoptysis.

26. Heavy proteinuria of more than 5 g per day (nephrotic syndrome) is associated with

a. Elevated serum cholesterol
b. Frothy urine
c. Elevation of the JVP
d. Pleural effusions
e. Lymphoedema

27. The following are recognized causes of nephrotic syndrome:

a. Mercury poisoning **syndrome:**
b. Systemic lupus erythematosus
c. Multiple myeloma
d. Malaria
e. Chronic pyelonephritis

28. In the nephrotic syndrome

a. Children have a worse prognosis than adults.
b. There is a recognized association with malignant tumours.
c. Pruritus is a characteristic feature.
d. Postural hypotension suggests amyloidosis.
e. Minimal lesion disease typically responds well to corticosteroids.

Answers overleaf

24. (*a, c, d*)
Haematuria is seen in many diseases of the renal system; however, it is not a typical feature of prostatic carcinoma or the relatively common congenital defect of duplex kidney.

25. (*b, e*)
Goodpasture's syndrome is associated with basement membrane antibodies which are thought to cross-react with pulmonary capillaries, the resultant damage producing haemoptysis. This syndrome usually runs a fulminant course and requires urgent treatment. Erythema nodosum is not a feature of Goodpasture's syndrome.

26. (*a, b, d*)
The heavy protein loss from nephrotic syndrome may result in frothy urine, low serum albumin, oedema (not lymphoedema) and pleural effusions. The elevated cholesterol and other plasma lipid components is thought to be related to low serum albumin concentration. The JVP is usually not elevated as the circulating vascular volume tends to be low.

27. (*a, b, c, d*)
Chronic pyelonephritis is not a cause of nephrotic syndrome.

28. (*b, d, e*)
Children generally have a better prognosis than adults, particularly when the histology shows 'minimal lesion' changes (approx. 80 per cent respond to corticosteroids against 20 per cent in adults). Tumours are a recognized cause of the syndrome. Amyloidosis, another cause of nephrotic syndrome, may present with postural hypotension due to autonomic neuropathy.

29. Acute tubular necrosis

a. Is associated with severe haemorrhage.
b. Almost never recovers.
c. Produces slight reduction in urine volume.
d. Is associated with severe crush injuries.
e. Is associated with a high urea content in the urine.

30. A diagnosis of renal artery stenosis is supported by the following:

a. Nephrotic syndrome
b. Abdominal bruit
c. Severe systemic hypertension
d. Loin pain
e. Haematuria

31. Pyelonephritis

a. Is most commonly caused by Klebsiella urinary infections.
b. Can exist without clinical symptoms.
c. Fever is rarely associated with rigors.
d. Typically causes clubbing of the pelvic calices.
e. Is associated with red cell casts in the urine.

32. Which of the following statements about renal tuberculosis are correct?

a. The primary renal lesion is typically in the renal papillae.
b. Pyuria is characteristic.
c. Haematuria is a recognized presentation.
d. Marked weight loss is a characteristic feature.
e. In men associated epididymal tuberculous lesions are typical.

33. Urinary calculi are

a. Most commonly composed of uric acid.
b. Associated with haematuria.
c. A recognized complication of prolonged immobilization.
d. One of the causes of hydronephrosis.
e. A recognized cause of pyelonephritis.

Answers overleaf

29. (*a, d*)
Acute tubular necrosis usually occurs after haemorrhagic shock particularly with crush injuries. It causes severe oliguria, any urine having a low urea content. Recovery tends to occur after about 10 days.

30. (*b, c*)
Renal artery stenosis is one of the causes of systemic arterial hypertension. An abdominal bruit is heard on rare occasions.

31. (*b, d*)
Chronic pyelonephritis is most commonly caused by *E. coli* infections and may exist without symptoms. Rigors are characteristic and the urine may contain leucocyte casts. Clubbing of the renal pelvic calices is a radiological feature of the condition.

32. (*b, c, e*)
The primary lesion in the kidney is cortical but is asymptomatic until the renal pelvis is involved. Pyuria is characteristic and haematuria may be present. Constitutional symptoms are not common and in men other parts of the genital tract are often affected.

33. (*b, c, d, e*)
The commonest constituent of renal calculi is calcium oxalate and one predisposing cause is prolonged immobilization. Stones may be complicated by hydronephrosis and pylonephritis if impacted at the pelvi-ureteric junction.

34. The causes of a large renal mass include

a. Hydronephrosis
b. Glomerulonephritis
c. Polycystic kidneys
d. Renal vein thrombosis
e. Hypernephroma

35. Which of the following statements about the bladder are correct?

a. Recurrent cystitis is commoner in men.
b. There is an association between bladder diverticuli and bladder calculi.
c. Prostatic enlargement is associated with nocturia.
d. Tumour of the bladder typically presents with haematuria.
e. Pain is a prominent feature of chronic urinary retention.

Answers overleaf

34. (*a, c, e*)
Renal vein thrombosis and glomerulonephritis are not causes of a renal mass; in fact, chronic glomerulonephritis may result in a small kidney.

35. (*b, c, d*)
Cystitis is much commoner in women. Pain is a prominent feature of acute rather than chronic retention, which is sometimes almost symptomless until renal failure develops.

1. A 10-year-old boy complains of backache and general tiredness. He is found to have smoky discoloration of his urine, facial oedema and papilloedema.

a. What is the likely diagnosis?
b. What is the cause of the papilloedema?
c. Name three abnormalities that you would expect to find in his urine.

2. A 50-year-old man was admitted to hospital with a myocardial infarction and then had a cardiac arrest. Forty-eight hours after successful resuscitation he had only passed 150 ml of urine. He had no abdominal pain and his bladder was not palpable.

a. What is the probable cause for the anuria?
b. What are the likely sequence of events over the next 2 weeks?

3. A 45-year-old man complained of persistent urinary frequency and dysuria. On examination, he was found to have painless enlargement of the epididymis. The urine contained significant numbers of pus cells, but no organisms were grown on routine culture.

a. What is the most likely diagnosis?
b. Give three relevant investigations.

4. A previously fit 64-year-old woman suddenly developed severe intermittent abdominal and loin pain. When examined, she was rolling from side to side in agony and had vomited several times.

a. What is the pain called and due to?
b. Name three diseases associated with this condition.

5. An elderly man was taken to casualty after being found collapsed at home. On examination, he was hyperventilating but there were no other abnormal respiratory signs. He had extensive bruising and his blood pressure was 200/115 mm. He subsequently had a grand mal convulsion.

a. Give the most likely cause for this clinical picture.
b. Why was he hyperventilating?
c. List two other clinical signs which may be present.

Answers overleaf

1. *a*. Acute glomerulonephritis
b. Systemic hypertension
c. (i) Blood
(ii) Protein
(iii) Granular casts

2. *a*. Acute tubular necrosis
b. Anuria and uraemic symptoms usually lasting up to 3 weeks followed by a diuretic recovery phase

3. *a*. Genitorenal tuberculosis
b. (i) Three early morning urine specimens for acid-fast bacilli
(ii) Chest X-ray for signs of old pulmonary involvement
(iii) Plain abdominal X-ray for renal calcification
(iv) Intravenous pyelogram

4. *a*. (i) Renal colic
(ii) Renal calculi
b. (i) Hyperparathyroidism
(ii) Gout
(iii) Cystineuria

5. *a*. Chronic renal failure
b. Because of a metabolic acidosis (Kussmaul's breathing)
c. (i) Pallor
(ii) Pitting oedema
(iii) Ammoniacal foetor

Arrange the following associations into their correct pairs:

1.	*A*. Polyuria	*a*. Retroperitoneal fibrosis
	B. Retention of urine	*b*. Cystitis
	C. Cough incontinence	*c*. Diabetes insipidus
	D. Oliguria	*d*. Prolapsed uterus
	E. Strangury	*e*. Traumatic paraplegia
2.	*A*. Severe abdominal pain	*a*. Hypertension
	B. Chest pain	*b*. Metabolic acidosis
	C. Papilloedema	*c*. Renal stones
	D. Peripheral oedema	*d*. Hypo-albuminaemia
	E. Kussmaul's breathing	*e*. Uraemic pericarditis
3.	*A*. Subperiosteal resorption of terminal phalanges	*a*. Hypernephroma
	B. Pseudo-fractures	*b*. Hyperparathyroidism
	C. Palpable kidney	*c*. Diabetes mellitus
	D. Posterior scrotal sinus	*d*. Osteomalacia
	E. Pruritus vulvae	*e*. Tuberculosis
4.	*A*. Smoky urine	*a*. Eating beetroot
	B. Pink urine	*b*. Alkaptonuria
	C. Red urine on standing	*c*. Acute glomerulonephritis
	D. Dark greenish/orange urine	*d*. Obstructive jaundice
	E. Black urine	*e*. Porphyria
5.	*A*. Glycosuria	*a*. Ehrlich reagent
	B. Haematuria	*b*. Nitroprusside reaction
	C. Proteinuria	*c*. Benedict's solution
	D. Urobilinogen	*d*. Buffered tetrabromphenol blue
	E. Ketoneuria	*e*. Orthotolidine oxidation
6.	*A*. Pneumaturia	*a*. Multiple myeloma
	B. Painless haematuria	*b*. Pyelonephritis
	C. Leucocyte casts	*c*. Vesicocolonic fistula
	D. Bence Jones proteinuria	*d*. Hypernephroma
	E. Calculi	*e*. Cystinuria

Answers overleaf

1. *A*......*c*
B......*e*
C......*d*
D......*a*
E......*b*

2. *A*......*c*
B......*e*
C......*a*
D......*d*
E......*b*

3. *A*......*b*
B......*d*
C......*a*
D......*e*
E......*c*

4. *A*......*c*
B......*a*
C......*e*
D......*d*
E......*b*

5. *A*......*c*
B......*e*
C......*d*
D......*a*
E......*b*

6. *A*......*c*
B......*d*
C......*b*
D......*a*
E......*e*

7. *A*. Streptococcal throat infection
B. Malignancy
C. Haemoptysis
D. Crush injury
E. Abdominal bruit

a. Goodpasture's syndrome
b. Renal artery stenosis
c. Nephrotic syndrome
d. Acute glomerulonephritis
e. Acute tubular necrosis

8. *A*. Renal mass
B. Chronic urinary retention
C. Epididymal mass
D. Papillary necrosis
E. Renal vein thrombosis

a. Tuberculosis
b. Chronic phenacetin administration
c. Nephrotic syndrome
d. Prostatic enlargement
e. Polycystic kidney

Answers overleaf

7. *A*......*d*
B......*c*
C......*a*
D......*e*
E......*b*

8. *A*......*e*
B......*d*
C......*a*
D......*b*
E......*c*

The Respiratory System

(Refer to Chapter 6 in *Symptoms and Signs in Clinical Medicine*, 11th edition, p. 159.)

1. Which of the following statements concerning cough are correct?

a. A 'brassy' cough is a characteristic feature of chronic bronchitis.
b. Fractured ribs are a recognized complication of severe coughing.
c. Cough syncope is caused by sudden reduction of arterial oxygen saturation.
d. A 'bovine' cough is typical of severe asthma.
e. Dry non-productive cough is characteristic of irritant dusts.

2. Nocturnal cough is typical of

a. Asthma
b. Pulmonary oedema
c. Gastro-oesophageal regurgitation
d. Chronic sinusitis
e. Kyphoscoliosis

3. Large quantity of sputum is a recognized feature of

a. Bronchiectasis
b. Asthma
c. Lung abscess
d. Empyema
e. Alveolar cell carcinoma

4. Sputum

a. Resembling anchovy sauce is typical of pulmonary hydatid disease.
b. Containing bronchial casts is characteristic of broncho-pulmonary aspergillosis.
c. Which is pink and frothy is typical of pulmonary oedema.
d. Consisting of pure pus is a complication of empyema.
e. Coloured yellow is always due to infection.

5. Which of the following are recognized causes of haemoptysis?

a. Tuberculosis
b. Mitral stenosis
c. Pulmonary infarction
d. Goodpasture's syndrome
e. Closed chest trauma (without rib fracture)

Answers overleaf

1. (*b, e*)
A 'brassy' cough is a feature of tracheal narrowing, while a 'bovine' cough is due to vocal cord paralysis. A non-productive cough occurs with irritant dusts, interstitial pulmonary fibrosis and some cases of asthma and infections. Two complications of severe coughing, particularly in elderly patients, are hair-line fractures of the ribs (cough fractures) and cough syncope in which increased intrathoracic pressure during coughing prevents venous return to the heart.

2. (*a, b, c, d*)
The recumbent posture is associated with nocturnal cough in cardiac failure, chronic sinusitis and gastro-oesophageal reflux. The reason why asthma is usually more troublesome at night is unknown.

3. (*a, c, d, e*)
Large quantities of purulent sputum are characteristic of bronchiectasis; other causes include lung abscess and empyema which have ruptured into the bronchial tree. Large amounts of thin watery sputum are a feature of some cases of alveolar cell carcinoma.

4. (*b, c, d*)
Rupture of an abscess or empyema into the bronchial tree usually results in the expectoration of pure pus (in the case of an amoebic abscess this resembles anchovy sauce). Bronchial casts are seen in asthma, particularly if it is complicated by bronchopulmonary aspergillosis. Pink frothy sputum is a classic symptom of severe pulmonary oedema. Although yellow discoloration of sputum is usually secondary to infection, large numbers of eosinophils may give a similar appearance.

5. (All correct)
Haemoptysis is a feature of all these conditions.

6. The following are highly suggestive of haemoptysis rather than haematemesis

a. Blood mixed with air
b. pH of 4·0
c. Dark red or brown blood from the onset of symptoms
d. Persistent small blood loss over many days
e. Cough preceding blood

7. Which of the following statements concerning dyspnoea are correct?

a. Narrowing of major airways rarely causes dyspnoea.
b. Acute renal failure is a recognized cause of severe dyspnoea.
c. Increased stiffness of the lungs results in dyspnoea.
d. Dyspnoea after exercise is typical of bronchial asthma.
e. Thyrotoxicosis is a recognized cause of dyspnoea.

8. Which of the following statements about different types of dyspnoea are correct?

a. Cheyne–Stokes breathing is normal in an awake 80-year-old.
b. Orthopnoea is occasionally made worse on standing.
c. Sighing respiration is a recognized feature of psychogenic dyspnoea.
d. Paroxysmal nocturnal dyspnoea is relieved by lying flat.
e. Effort dyspnoea after mild exercise only occurs in the presence of respiratory or cardiac disease.

9. Pain

a. When pleuritic arises from pain receptors in the visceral pleura.
b. Arising from the diaphragm is typically referred to 1st and 2nd cervical dermatomes.
c. From pulmonary pain receptors has a dull and aching character.
d. When pleuritic almost never radiates to the abdomen.
e. From a Pancoast tumour (carcinoma arising in lung apex) is typically felt in the arm.

Answers overleaf

6. (*a, d, e*)
At times it can be very difficult to distinguish between haemoptysis and haematemesis. The principal features in favour of the former are a cough preceding any blood, blood mixed with air and small quantities of bright red blood which continues for several days. A very acid pH is typical of haematemesis.

7. (*b, c, d, e*)
Dyspnoea is a subjective symptom and has numerous causes. Narrowing of the airways as in asthma is a common cause and this may only be present after exercise (exercise-induced asthma). Increased stiffness of the lungs (reduced compliance) for any reason is another cause (e.g. pulmonary oedema or cryptogenic fibrosing alveolitis). Metabolic acidosis and thyrotoxicosis produce dyspnoea by stimulation of the respiratory centre.

8. (*c*)
Cheyne–Stokes respiration is almost always a sign of grave illness. Orthopnoea by definition occurs only on lying flat and paroxysmal nocturnal dyspnoea is relieved by sitting or standing. Effort dyspnoea is usually due to respiratory or cardiac disease, but may occur with other conditions such as anaemia, thyrotoxicosis and psychological illnesses (when sighing respirations are often observed).

9. (*e*)
Pleuritic pain arises from the parietal pleura, the visceral pleura and lung parenchyma being insensitive to pain. Pain from the central part of the diaphragm arises from the phrenic nerve (3rd and 4th cervical segments) and is often referred to the shoulder tip. Chest pain also commonly radiates to the abdomen and back, and in the case of a Pancoast tumour to the arm.

10. Extrathoracic manifestations of respiratory diseases include

a. Tremors
b. Lassitude
c. Night sweats
d. Myopathy
e. Convulsions

11. Cyanosis

a. Occurs when 10 per cent of total haemoglobin is desaturated.
b. Is not recognized until the arterial PO_2 is below 10·6 kPa.
c. When peripheral is a typical feature of mitral stenosis.
d. Due to cold is most marked on the tongue.
e. Is a prominent feature of left-to-right shunts.

12. Central cyanosis commonly accompanies

a. Pneumonia
b. Polycythaemia
c. Uncomplicated atrial septal defect
d. Fibrosing alveolitis
e. Bronchial carcinoma

13. Enterogenous cyanosis (due to abnormal pigments) is caused by

a. Ingestion of shell fish
b. Sulphonamide drugs
c. Analgesics
d. Poisoning with methylated spirit
e. Presence of haemoglobin M (hereditary haemoglobinopathy)

14. Cyanosis may be abolished by oxygen therapy in the following circumstances:

a. Right-to-left shunt
b. Chronic bronchitis
c. Polycythaemia
d. Enterogenous cyanosis
e. Pneumonia

Answers overleaf

10. (All correct)
Tremor, convulsions and sweating are features of carbon dioxide retention (hypercarbia). Severe night sweats are seen with tuberculosis. Myopathy is a rare complication of bronchial carcinoma.

11. (*b, c*)
Cyanosis is diagnosed when 5 g/dl (30 per cent) of total haemoglobin in the capillaries is desaturated. This only occurs when the oxygen tension has fallen to below 10·6 kPa. In peripheral cyanosis (e.g. due to cold or mitral stenosis) the tongue is a normal colour. Central cyanosis is a feature of right-to-left (not left-to-right) shunts.

12. (*a, b, d, e*)
Central cyanosis, in which the blood in the aorta is desaturated, is a feature of inadequate pulmonary perfusion of ventilated areas (e.g. pneumonia and bronchial neoplasms), impaired oxygen transfer through lung tissue (e.g. fibrosing alveolitis), normal percentage saturation but increase in the absolute unsaturated haemoglobin concentration (polycythaemia), right-to-left shunts and abnormal haemoglobin pigments (enterogenous cyanosis).

13. (*b, c, e*)
Enterogenous cyanosis is due to abnormal pigments (methaemoglobin or sulphaemoglobin) in the blood. Causes include various drugs (analgesics and sulphonamides), chemicals and hereditary defects (hereditary methaemoglobinaemia due to either enzyme deficiency or haemoglobin-M).

14. (*b, c, e*)
Oxygen therapy abolishes central cyanosis unless there are abnormal haemoglobin pigments or a right-to-left shunt bypassing the heart is present.

23. Which of the following statements regarding the lungs are correct?

a. The right middle lobe bronchus arises from the anterior wall of the bronchus intermedius.
b. The left middle lobe has two main divisions.
c. The left main bronchus is almost in line with the trachea.
d. The membranous portion of the trachea is anterior.
e. The right upper lobe has three main divisions.

24. Vocal fremitus is reduced over the lower zones with

a. Pleural effusions
b. Collapse of a lung secondary to bronchial blockage
c. Consolidation
d. Pneumothorax
e. Chronic bronchitis

25. Which of the following statements about percussion are correct?

a. The striking finger should be at 45° to the finger on the chest wall.
b. Light percussion gives information about superficial lung tissue.
c. The percussed finger should always be placed in a rib interspace.
d. Only the pulp of the percussed finger should be in contact with the chest wall.
e. The striking finger should be moved from the metacarpo-phalangeal joints.

26. Causes of a dull percussion note include

a. Pneumothorax
b. Pneumonia
c. Pleural effusion
d. Emphysema
e. Pleural thickening

Answers overleaf

23. (*a, e*)
The right middle lobe bronchus arises anteriorly, while on the left there is no middle lobe. The right not left main bronchus is in line with the trachea and is thus the most likely site for impaction of a foreign body. The membranous portion of the trachea is posterior and the right upper lobe has three divisions (apical, posterior and anterior).

24. (*a, b, d*)
Vocal fremitus is decreased with pleural effusions, lung collapse and pneumothorax. It is increased in consolidation and normal in chronic bronchitis.

25. (*b*)
Percussion is performed with the striking finger kept at 90°, the movement being from the wrist. The percussed finger should be flat on the chest wall and it does not matter whether it overlies a rib or intercostal space. Light percussion sets superficial and heavy percussion deep structures into vibration.

26. (*b, c, e*)
A dull percussion note is found when the underlying tissue is solid (e.g. consolidation and pleural thickening), or in the presence of fluid. Pneumothorax and emphysema are causes of hyper-resonance.

27. Which of the following statements about breathing sounds heard at the mouth are correct?

a. Wheezing is due to narrowing of small airways (less than 2 mm).
b. Stridor is caused by narrowing of subsegmental bronchi.
c. Kussmaul's breathing is characteristic of salicylate poisoning.
d. Rattling breathing is typically associated with poor cough reflex.
e. Stertorous breathing is a feature of coma.

28. Breath sounds

a. Are reduced on the side on which the patient is lying.
b. When 'vesicular' are due to air rushing into the alveoli.
c. Of a bronchial nature are always abnormal at the lung bases.
d. Are softer in children than adults (puerile breathing).
e. With a 'cog-wheel' character occur in nervous people.

29. Diminished breath sounds are characteristic of

a. Pleural fluid
b. Bronchiectasis
c. Emphysema
d. Pneumothorax
e. Carcinoma with bronchial occlusion

30. Which of the following are characteristically associated with bronchial breathing?

a. No gap between inspiration and expiration
b. Presence of high-frequency sounds
c. Expiration shorter than inspiration
d. Patent major airways
e. Whispering pectoriloquy

31. Typical causes of bronchial breathing include

a. Consolidation of the lung
b. Severe pulmonary oedema
c. Collapse of the right lower lobe
d. Pleural tumours
e. Cryptogenic fibrosing alveolitis

Answers overleaf

27. (*c, d, e*)
Wheezing typically arises from narrowing of larger airways (air flow in very small airways is generally not sufficient to induce wheezing). Stridor is a characteristic low-pitched wheezing sound which is due to narrowing in the trachea or larynx. Kussmaul's breathing has a hissing quality and is due to hyperventilation through an almost closed mouth (*see* Question 20). Stertorous breathing, due to vibrations of soft tissues in the nasopharynx, occurs in coma and some normal people during sleep. Rattling respiration is associated with a poor cough reflex and is often heard in elderly patients with bronchopneumonia.

28. (*a, c, e*)
Breath sounds are thought to arise in the larger bronchi (turbulent air flow), the high-frequency components being filtered out as the sound traverses the lung tissue. Such sounds are louder in children (puerile breathing) and reduced on the side on which a patient is lying. 'Bronchovesicular' breathing is harsh and normal at the apices and in the interscapular regions but not at the bases. 'Cog-wheel' breathing is typically present in nervous patients.

29. (*a, c, d, e*)
Diminished breath sounds are characteristic of all these conditions with the exception of bronchiectasis.

30. (*b, d, e*)
Bronchial breathing has a similar quality to tracheal breath sounds, inspiration and expiration being of the same intensity and duration and separated by a pause. High as well as low frequencies are transmitted through consolidated lung, giving the sound its clarity and producing the phenomenon of whispering pectoriloquy. Major airways are usually, but not invariably, patent as sound can enter directly from the trachea into collapsed upper lobes.

31. (*a*)
Bronchial breathing is associated with consolidation (and occasionally with collapse of the upper lobe), but not typically with pulmonary oedema, pleural tumours, collapse of lower lobes or fibrosing alveolitis.

32. Amphoric breathing

a. Is heard over a tuberculous cavity.
b. Is associated with a gap between inspiration and expiration.
c. Has a 'hollow' sound quality.
d. Is typically present over a communicating pneumothorax.
e. Is a characteristic finding over a pneumonectomy space.

33. Which of the following statements regarding vocal resonance are correct?

a. Normal lung filters out low-frequency sound.
b. Vocal resonance is louder in men than women.
c. Whispering pectoriloquy is very occasionally present over the lower lobes in normal, very thin people.
d. Aegophony is heard at the base of a pleural effusion.
e. Bronchophony is heard over consolidated lung.

34. Wheezing

a. Characteristically depends on a resonating column of air within a bronchus.
b. When high pitched, is characteristic of a carcinomatous bronchial stricture.
c. If fixed and monophonic, is typical of bronchial asthma.
d. Is typically more marked on inspiration.
e. Is not a feature of emphysema.

35. A pleural friction rub

a. Is absent in the presence of a pleural effusion.
b. Occurs only on inspiration.
c. May be palpable.
d. Is transiently abolished by coughing.
e. Is characteristically associated with a severe continuous ache over the affected area.

Answers overleaf

32. (*a, b, c, d*)
Amphoric breathing is a type of bronchial breathing which has a 'hollow' quality and is heard when a cavity is communicating with a large bronchus. The classic cause was a tuberculous cavity, but it is now more often heard over a communicating pneumothorax. It is not present over a pneumonectomy space unless the bronchial stump breaks down.

33. (*e*)
Normal lung tissue filters out high- (not low-) frequency sound. Whispering pectoriloquy is never present over normal lungs and aegophony is heard over the top of a pleural effusion. Increased vocal resonance (bronchophony) is heard over consolidated lung because it conducts sound better than normal air containing lung tissue.

34. (All incorrect)
Wheezing is due to vibration of lung tissue and is largely independent of the resonating column of air within a bronchus. It is common in any cause of airflow obstruction (including emphysema) and tends to be most marked on expiration. A high-pitched wheeze is typical of asthma and a fixed monophonic wheeze of carcinomatous stricture.

35. (*c*)
A pleural rub is often heard in the presence of fluid and may occasionally be palpable. It is associated with sharp stabbing pain (pleurisy) which is made worse on inspiration and coughing.

36. Crackles

a. Are mainly due to air bubbling through fluid in the bronchi.
b. If early in inspiration, are suggestive of chronic bronchitis.
c. Are more often present at the lung apices than bases.
d. Due to fibrosing alveolitis, are transiently abolished by coughing.
e. When present with pulmonary oedema, signify intra-alveolar oedema.

37. Bronchial asthma

a. Is associated with infantile eczema.
b. When occurring for the first time in middle age, is typically associated with multiple skin-prick allergies (atopy).
c. Is least troublesome in the early hours of the morning.
d. Does not run in families.
e. May produce permanent chest-wall deformities.

38. Which of the following statements about chronic bronchitis are correct?

a. The diagnostic features are cough and wheeze.
b. May be complicated by signs of right-heart failure.
c. The respiratory centre typically becomes less sensitive to hypercarbia.
d. Sputum production is most marked first thing in the morning.
e. Finger clubbing is a recognized feature.

39. Recognized features of bronchiectasis include

a. Increased prevalence in the lower lobes
b. Cystic changes on the chest X-ray
c. Small amounts of watery sputum
d. Coarse inspiratory crackles
e. *Haemophilus influenzae* infections

40. Recognized causes of bronchiectasis include

a. Whooping cough
b. Pneumonia
c. Pulmonary tuberculosis
d. Rheumatoid disease
e. Cystic fibrosis

Answers overleaf

36. (*b*)
Crackles most commonly occur in conditions associated with stiffness of the lungs (e.g. fibrosing alveolitis, pulmonary oedema and pneumonia). It is thought that in these circumstances smaller airways close on expiration and when they snap open during inspiration the sudden equalization of pressure across the airways results in crackling sounds. Crackles are most commonly heard at the lung bases, and tend to be early in inspiration in chronic bronchitis and late in pulmonary oedema and alveolitis.

37. (*a, e*)
Extrinsic asthma, which frequently runs in families, is often accompanied by infantile eczema and multiple skin-prick allergies (atopy). Intrinsic (adult onset) asthma is not typically associated with atopy but, like extrinsic asthma, it is often worse in the early hours of the morning. If childhood asthma is severe, it may result in pigeon-chest deformity.

38. (*b, c, d*)
The diagnostic feature of chronic bronchitis is a chronic productive cough which is worse in the morning and during winter months. In later stages it is frequently complicated by signs of right-heart failure and the respiratory centre becomes less sensitive to hypercarbia. Finger clubbing is not a feature of this condition and, if present, may signify the development of a bronchial neoplasm.

39. (*a, b, d, e*)
The chief symptom of bronchiectasis is expectoration of large quantities of purulent sputum which is often infected with *Haemophilus influenzae*. It most commonly affects the lower lobes and hence the typical coarse early to mid-inspiratory crackles are most often heard over the lower zones. The chest radiograph may show cystic changes.

40. (All correct)
Bronchiectasis most commonly results from severe childhood pneumonia, but there are many other causes including all those mentioned in this question.

41. Which of the following are recognized features of pulmonary oedema?

a. Wheezing
b. End-inspiratory crackles
c. Orthopnoea
d. Viscid sputum
e. Haemoptysis

42. Causes of pulmonary oedema include

a. Mitral stenosis
b. Nitric oxide inhalation
c. Pneumonia
d. Asbestos dust inhalation
e. Phosgene gas inhalation

43. Which of the following are characteristic features of consolidation?

a. Decreased movement over the affected hemithorax
b. Inspiratory crackles
c. Decreased tactile vocal fremitus
d. Marked displacement of the trachea
e. Kussmaul's respiration

44. Typical causes of consolidation include

a. Tuberculosis
b. Pneumonia
c. Pulmonary infarction
d. Chronic bronchitis
e. Sarcoidosis

45. Absorption pulmonary collapse is associated with

a. Bronchial asthma
b. Inhalation of a foreign body
c. Childhood pulmonary tuberculosis
d. Pleural effusion
e. Carcinoma of the bronchus

Answers overleaf

41. (*a, b, c, e*)
Orthopnoea is a common symptom of pulmonary oedema due to increased pulmonary congestion on lying flat. Less common symptoms include wheezing and blood-tinged watery sputum. End-inspiratory crackles are a characteristic sign resulting from increased stiffness of the lungs.

42. (*a, b, c, e*)
The commonest cause of pulmonary oedema is cardiac disease (e.g. ischaemic or valvular heart disease). It can also occur with pneumonia and inhalation of irritant gases (e.g. phosgene and nitric oxide). Asbestos dust is not a cause.

43. (*a, b*)
Consolidation is associated with reduced movement over the affected hemithorax, dull percussion note and increased tactile vocal fremitus (the latter due to the good transmission through consolidated lung tissue). The trachea is not displaced unless there is coexistant collapse. Auscultation usually reveals bronchial breathing and inspiratory crackles. Kussmaul's respiration is a feature of metabolic acidosis.

44. (*a, b, c*)
Typical causes of consolidation are acute infections, tuberculosis, bronchial neoplasms and pulmonary infarction. Uncomplicated chronic bronchitis and sarcoidosis are not causes.

45. (*a, b, c, e*)
All these are causes of pulmonary collapse; however, pleural effusion typically produces compression not absorption collapse.

46. Extensive absorption collapse is typically associated with the following physical signs:

a. Bronchial breathing if the upper lobes are involved
b. Dull percussion note
c. Displacement of the apex beat
d. Increased breath sounds over the affected area
e. Cavernous breathing

47. Which of the following are typical manifestations of early fibrosing alveolitis?

a. Showers of early inspiratory crackles
b. Finger clubbing
c. Whispering pectoriloquy
d. Hypercarbia
e. Nasal polypi

48. Pleurisy is

a. Typically associated with grunting respiration
b. A recognized feature of rheumatoid disease
c. Sometimes associated with a palpable friction rub
d. A feature of pulmonary infarction
e. Typically associated with hyperventilation

49. Signs of a large pleural effusion include

a. Displacement of the trachea towards the effusion
b. Aegophony
c. Engorgement of the JVP
d. Barrel-shaped chest
e. Reduced vocal fremitus

50. Which of the following statements relating to pleural effusions are correct?

a. Mesothelioma is a common cause of chylous effusion.
b. An effusion with a protein content of 8 g/l is typical of heart failure.
c. Carcinomatous effusions are always blood-stained.
d. Empyema is more common in patients with rheumatoid disease.
e. Subphrenic abscess is a cause of sterile pleural effusion.

Answers overleaf

46. (*a, b, c*)
Collapse is associated with reduced chest movement and percussion note. Breath sounds are usually diminished or absent but may be bronchial over collapsed upper lobes (tracheal sounds being transmitted directly into the adjacent upper lobe). The mediastinum moves towards the side of the collapse. Cavernous breathing is a type of bronchial breathing heard over cavities.

47. (*b*)
Diffuse interstitial pulmonary fibrosis (due to fibrosing alveolitis) is associated with showers of late inspiratory crackles (as the condition progresses these tend to fill the whole of inspiration). Finger clubbing is common early and hypercarbia very late in the natural history of fibrosing alveolitis. Whispering pectoriloquy is a feature of consolidation not interstitial pulmonary fibrosis.

48. (*a, b, c, d*)
Pleuritic chest pain results in shallow respiration often accompanied by a grunting noise. The only physical sign is a pleural friction rub which may be palpable. Pleurisy is a feature of pulmonary infarction, pneumonia, pleural tumours and collagen diseases such as rheumatoid arthritis.

49. (*b, c, e*)
Pleural effusion is characteristically associated with reduced chest wall movement (barrel chest is seen in chronic airflow obstruction). The trachea is deviated away from the effusion and breath sounds and vocal fremitus are reduced. Occasionally at the top of a large effusion aegophony, a type of bronchial breathing, is heard. The JVP may be engorged with very large effusions.

50. (*d, e*)
Mesothelioma, like pleural carcinoma, usually but not invariably causes a blood-stained effusion. Chylous fluid is associated with damage to the thoracic duct. The effusion in heart failure is a transudate (low protein content). Empyema, both sterile and infective, is more common in rheumatoid disease. Another cause of pleural reaction, often with effusion or empyema, is subphrenic abscess.

51. Causes of pneumothorax include

a. Small subpleural bulla in young women
b. Perforated oesophagus
c. Diffuse interstitial pulmonary fibrosis
d. Tuberculosis
e. Childhood bronchial asthma

52. Which of the following are typical of pneumothorax?

a. Amphoric breath sounds and a closed pneumothorax
b. Hydropneumothorax and a curvilinear fluid level on the chest X-ray
c. Mediastinal emphysema and a 'clicking' sound (Hamman's sign)
d. Surgical emphysema
e. JVP engorgement and tension pneumothorax

53. Mediastinal obstruction is typically accompanied by

a. Third nerve palsy
b. Horner's syndrome
c. Stridor
d. Brassy cough
e. Headaches

54. Emphysema is associated with

a. More vertically placed ribs than normal
b. Prolonged inspiratory phase of breathing
c. Reduced cardiac dullness to percussion
d. Early development of cor pulmonale
e. Alpha-1 antitrypsin deficiency

55. Recognized complications of carcinoma of the bronchus include

a. Obstructive emphysema
b. Proximal muscle weakness
c. Hyponatraemia
d. Painful swelling of the ankles
e. Pleural effusion without mediastinal shift

Answers overleaf

51. (All correct)
These are all causes of pneumothorax. The commonest is a small subpleural bulla most often seen in men but also the commonest cause in women.

52. (*c, d, e*)
Amphoric breath sounds are occasionally heard over an open (communicating) pneumothorax which is acting as a large resonating cavity. Hydropneumothorax is characterized by a horizontal fluid level on the chest X-ray. Surgical emphysema and a clicking sound synchronous with the cardiac contractions are both features of mediastinal emphysema. When a pneumothorax is under tension, cardiac function becomes embarrassed and the JVP is engorged; if not relieved promptly this may be a fatal condition.

53. (*b, c, d, e*)
Mediastinal obstruction may be complicated by superior vena caval obstruction (this may result in severe headaches), Horner's syndrome, diaphragmatic paralysis, vocal cord paralysis, dyspnoea, stridor and dysphagia. A brassy cough due to a tumour pressing on the trachea and a bovine cough due to recurrent nerve paralysis are features of mediastinal obstruction; however, a 3rd nerve palsy is not caused by this condition.

54. (*c, e*)
Emphysema is typically associated with over-expansion of the lungs (barrel-shaped chest) which causes the ribs to be more horizontally placed. The breath sounds are reduced with a prolonged expiratory phase, percussion note is hyper-resonant and there is a reduction in the cardiac dullness. Cor pulmonale is a very late complication of primary emphysema and is more characteristic of chronic bronchitis. One rare cause of emphysema is alpha-1 antitrypsin deficiency.

55. (All correct)
Carcinoma of the bronchus may partially obstruct a major bronchus resulting in over-inflation of the lung beyond the obstruction (obstructive emphysema). Pleural effusion without mediastinal shift is a common association because of underlying collapse. Hyponatraemia may be caused by the tumour secreting antidiuretic hormone, and swellings of the feet and hands by pulmonary osteoarthropathy.

56. Which of the following are true?

a. Tomography involves the introduction of radio-opaque dye into the lungs.
b. Diaphragmatic movement is assessed by bronchography.
c. Ziehl–Neelsen's stain is used to demonstrate malignant cells in the sputum.
d. Angiography is usually the best way of demonstrating a small bronchial carcinoma.
e. A positive Mantoux test always indicates active tuberculosis.

57. The following pulmonary function tests are typically reduced in chronic obstructive bronchitis:

a. Forced expiratory volume in the first second (FEV 1)
b. $PaCO_2$
c. Forced vital capacity
d. Maximum voluntary ventilation
e. Residual volume

Answers overleaf

56. (All incorrect)

Tomography is a technique of focusing X-rays at different depths in the lungs. Bronchography is used to outline the airways by the introduction of dye into the bronchial tree (diaphragmatic movement is seen with screening). Angiography is not usually used to demonstrate bronchial carcinomas. A positive Mantoux test confirms previous exposure to tuberculosis (or BCG vaccination) but does not necessarily mean active disease; the only way to confirm this is by demonstrating the bacilli (most commonly by using Ziehl–Neelsen's stain).

57. (*a, c, d*)

Chronic airflow obstruction results in reduction of the FEV 1, peak expiratory flow rate and maximal voluntary ventilation. The forced vital capacity falls but not to the same extent as the FEV 1. The $Pa\text{CO}_2$ tends to rise because of hypoventilation and the residual volume is high because of air trapping.

1. An elderly man, a heavy smoker, with a long history of cough, sputum and wheezing dyspnoea on effort, presents with a morning occipital headache and vomiting of 2 months' duration.
a. Give two possible causes for the headaches and vomiting.
b. What physical sign is common to both these causes?

2. A 25-year-old married woman had a sudden transient attack of breathlessness, followed a few hours later by chest pain and haemoptysis. A pleural rub was heard on the right side and the pulmonary second sound was accentuated.
a. What is the most urgent condition to exclude?
b. List four additional questions which should be put to the patient.

3. A previously healthy teenage boy complains of sudden dyspnoea with sharp left-sided chest pain. On examination, the trachea is deviated to the right and the breath sounds are diminished over the left lung, but there are no other abnormal signs.
a. What is the diagnosis?
b. How might it be proved?

4. A 50-year-old woman complains of bursting headaches on lying and bending down. Examination reveals suffusion and oedema of the face.
a. What is the cause of these symptoms?
b. What is the most likely underlying diagnosis?
c. Name three other clinical signs which might be present.

5. A 66-year-old man presents with gradually increasing dyspnoea only on exercise. On examination he has a tachycardia of 104 beats/min but no other cardiovascular abnormality. There are showers of late inspiratory crackles over both lung bases. His ECG is normal.
a. Give the most likely diagnosis.
b. What might his occupation have been.
c. Name two other typical clinical features.

Answers overleaf

1. *a.* (i) Bronchial carcinoma with cerebral metastases
(ii) Chronic bronchitis with carbon dioxide retention
b. Papilloedema

2. *a.* Pulmonary embolism
b. (i) Any previous episodes of similar symptoms?
(ii) Any history of venous disorders in the legs?
(iii) Recent immobilization or major surgery (including childbirth)?
(iv) Is she taking the contraceptive pill?

3. *a.* Spontaneous pneumothorax
b. (i) Postero-anterior chest radiograph in expiration
(ii) By intubation and aspiration of air

4. *a.* Superior vena caval obstruction
b. Neoplasm involving the superior mediastinum (most commonly carcinoma of the bronchus)
c. (i) Engorged non-pulsatile jugular veins
(ii) Stridor
(iii) Hoarse voice

5. *a.* Diffuse interstitial pulmonary fibrosis (fibrosing alveolitis)
b. Asbestos worker
c. (i) Finger clubbing
(ii) Non-productive cough
(iii) Central cyanosis

6. An elderly man presents with severe dyspnoea. On examination, he is found to have poor movement of the left hemithorax, a central trachea, reduced air entry over the mid- and lower zones and a dull percussion note.

a. What is the explanation for these physical signs?
b. What do you think is the underlying diagnosis?
c. What two investigations should be performed?

Answers overleaf

6. *a*. Pleural effusion with underlying pulmonary collapse
b. Carcinoma of the bronchus with pleural secondary deposits
c. (i) Chest radiograph
(ii) Pleural aspiration

Arrange the following associations into their correct pairs:

1. *A*. Brassy cough
B. 'Anchovy sauce' sputum
C. Bovine cough
D. Bronchial casts in the sputum
E. Large quantities of sputum

a. Vocal cord paralysis
b. Aspergillosis
c. Alveolar cell carcinoma
d. Tracheal stenosis
e. Amoebic abscess

2. *A*. Proximal muscle weakness
B. Night sweats
C. Pursed-lip breathing
D. Kussmaul's breathing
E. Central cyanosis uncorrected by breathing oxygen

a. Emphysema
b. Right-to-left shunt
c. Acute renal failure
d. Carcinoma of bronchus
e. Pulmonary tuberculosis

3. *A*. Pigeon chest
B. Rib hump
C. Reduced tactile vocal fremitus
D. Tracheal tug
E. Stridor

a. Kyphoscoliosis
b. Childhood asthma
c. Retrosternal goitre
d. Pneumothorax
e. Aortic aneurysm

4. *A*. Amphoric breathing
B. Pleural friction
C. Late inspiratory crackles
D. Dull percussion note
E. Early inspiratory crackles

a. Chronic bronchitis
b. Communicating pneumothorax
c. Fibrosing alveolitis
d. Pulmonary embolism
e. Pleural thickening

5. *A*. Haemoptysis
B. Monophonic wheeze
C. Finger clubbing
D. Aegophony
E. Engorged non-pulsatile jugular vein

a. Large benign pleural effusion
b. Fibrosing alveolitis
c. Malignant thymoma
d. Mitral stenosis
e. Stenosis of a major bronchus

6. *A*. Painful swollen ankles
B. Surgical emphysema
C. Nasal polypi
D. Reduced cardiac dullness
E. Whispering pectoriloquy

a. Pneumonia
b. Asthma
c. Peripheral lung carcinoma
d. Ruptured oesophagus
e. Pulmonary emphysema

Answers overleaf

1. *A......d*
B......e
C......a
D......b
E......c

2. *A......d*
B......e
C......a
D......c
E......b

3. *A......b*
B......a
C......d
D......e
E......c

4. *A......b*
B......d
C......c
D......e
E......a

5. *A......d*
B......e
C......b
D......a
E......c

6. *A......c*
B......d
C......b
D......e
E......a

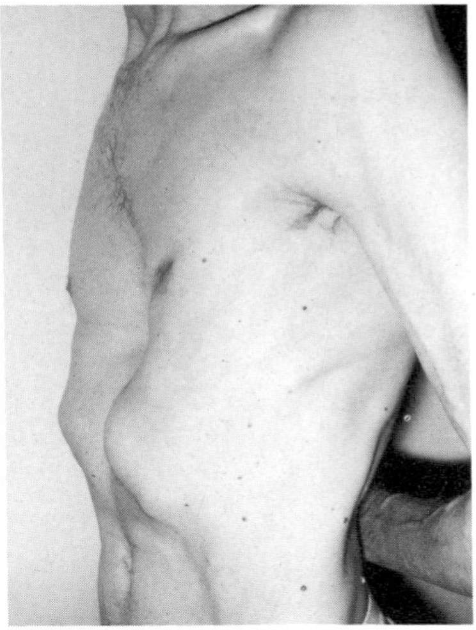

Fig. 6.1
a. What abnormality is shown?
b. What serious impact may this have on heart or lungs?

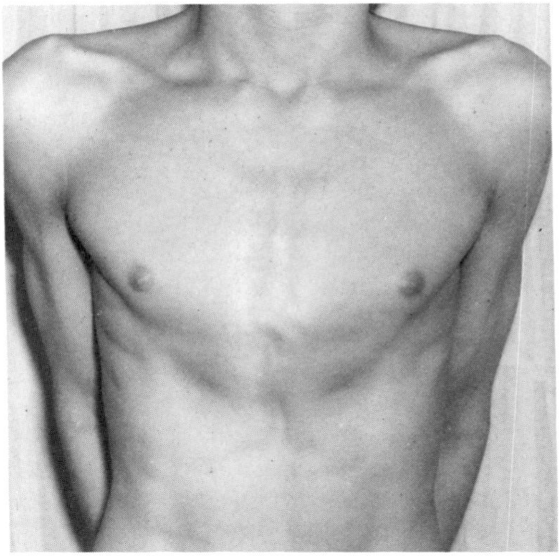

Fig. 6.2
a. Describe this appearance in English and in Latin.
b. Give two predisposing causes in childhood.

Answers overleaf

Fig. 6.1
a. Funnel sternum (pectus excavatum)
b. None

Fig. 6.2
a. Pigeon chest. Pectus carinatum
b. Rickets; asthma

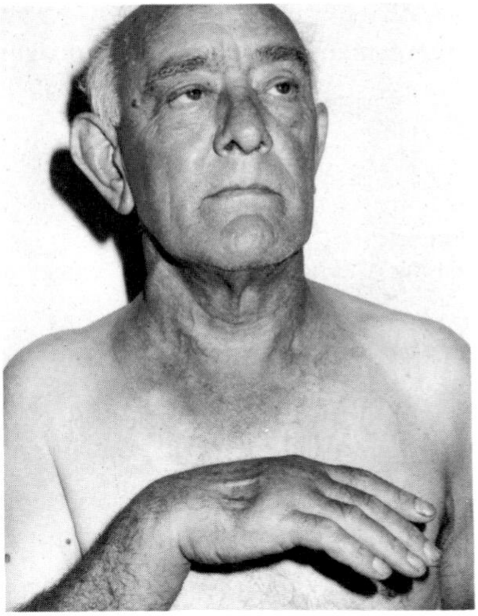

Fig. 6.3
a. List three abnormal signs shown.
b. Where is the site of the lesion?

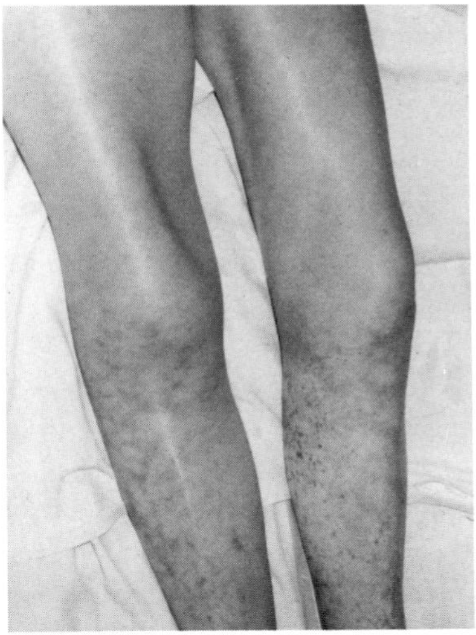

Fig. 6.4
a. Why does this patient have difficulty climbing the stairs?
b. Which three endocrine disorders may give rise to this appearance?

Answers overleaf

Fig. 6.3
a. Right-sided ptosis; jugular venous engorgement; pitting oedema of right hand
b. Right superior mediastinum

Fig. 6.4
a. Because of wasting of the quadriceps muscles.
b. Diabetes, hyperthyroidism and Cushing's syndrome can all cause a proximal myopathy.

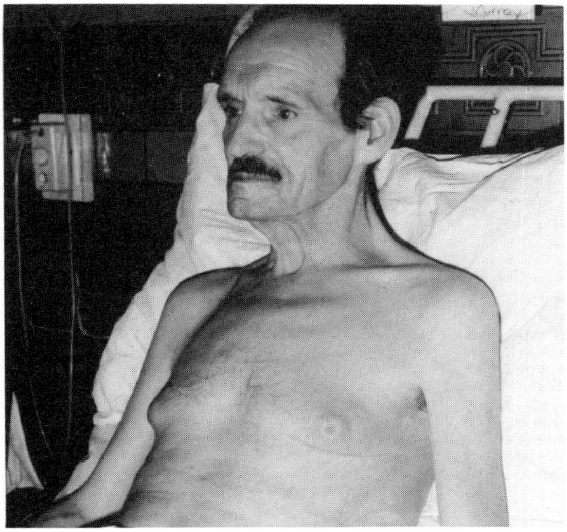

Fig. 6.5
List three drugs and one disease which might give rise to this appearance.

Answers overleaf

Fig. 6.5
Spironolactone; digoxin; oestrogen preparation; bronchial carcinoma

The Cardiovascular System

(Refer to Chapter 7 in *Symptoms and Signs in Clinical Medicine*, 11th edition, p. 201.)

1. **Which of the following statements about dyspnoea due to cardiac disease are correct?**
   a. It occurs as an early feature of aortic incompetence.
   b. Paroxysmal dyspnoea at rest may be confused with bronchial asthma.
   c. Orthopnoea occasionally occurs during walking exercise.
   d. Cheyne–Stokes breathing is pathognomonic of severe heart failure.
   e. Paroxysmal dyspnoea at rest is associated with a rise in left atrial pressure.

2. **Palpitations are always associated with**
   a. Hyperthyroidism
   b. Hypertension
   c. Anxiety
   d. Paroxysmal arrhythmias
   e. Pericarditis

3. **Ischaemic cardiac pain**
   a. Originates from nerves in the visceral pericardium.
   b. Is a recognized feature of aortic valve disease.
   c. Is sometimes felt in the jaw and neck.
   d. Is characteristically made worse by rest.
   e. Is always present following myocardial infarction.

4. **Precordial pain is a recognized feature of**
   a. Anxiety
   b. Pleurisy
   c. Oesophagitis
   d. Costochondritis (Tietze's syndrome)
   e. Pericarditis

5. **Untreated congestive heart failure is associated with**
   a. Right hypochondrial pain
   b. Haemoptysis
   c. Oliguria
   d. Psychological changes
   e. Anorexia

Answers overleaf

1. (*b, e*)
Aortic incompetence, unlike mitral stenosis, rarely causes dyspnoea in its early stages. Paroxysmal dyspnoea at rest is occasionally associated with wheezing and in these circumstances can be confused with bronchial asthma, while orthopnoea (by definition) can only occur when lying down. Cheyne–Stokes breathing is associated with cerebral haemorrhage, meningitis and advanced uraemia as well as severe heart failure. A rise in left atrial pressure is characteristic of dyspnoea due to pulmonary congestion.

2. (All incorrect)
Palpitation (awareness of the heart beating) is very common in anxious people and is often associated with extra systoles. Patients with a tachycardia due to heart disease are frequently unaware of the heart's action.

3. (*b, c*)
Cardiac pain originates from either the myocardial or the parietal pericardial nerves, the visceral pericardium being insensitive. These nerves originate from the upper four or five thoracic spinal segments and hence the pain may be referred to the neck, jaws or arms. It is made worse by exercise, not rest, and is associated with aortic valve disease. Paradoxically pain is not always a feature of myocardial infarction particularly in elderly patients.

4. (All correct)
All these factors are associated with precordial pain. Oesophageal pain can be particularly difficult to distinguish from cardiac pain as the lower oesophagus has a similar segmental innervation to the heart.

5. (All correct)
Untreated cardiac failure results in the liver and gastrointestinal tract being engorged with blood causing anorexia and right hypochondrial pain due to stretching of the liver capsule. Sluggish blood flow in this condition also causes poor renal perfusion resulting in oliguria and contributes to the psychological changes.

6. Syncope is a recognized feature of

a. Paroxysmal tachycardia
b. Complete heart block
c. Coarctation of the aorta
d. Aortic stenosis
e. Atrial myxoma

7. Pitting oedema is characteristically seen in

a. Lymphoedema
b. Hypoproteinaemia
c. Idiopathic portal vein thrombosis
d. Unilateral renal artery stenosis
e. Myxoedema

8. Cyanosis is characteristically seen

a. When 2 g/dl of capillary blood is desaturated
b. In Fallot's tetralogy
c. In atrial septal defects associated with severe pulmonary hypertension
d. In large pulmonary arteriovenous shunts
e. In mitral stenosis

9. Pulsation in the epigastrium is a recognized feature of

a. Normal people
b. Tricuspid incompetence
c. Hypertrophy of the heart
d. Abdominal aortic aneurysm
e. Uncomplicated coarctation of the aorta

10. Which of the following statements about the pulse are correct?

a. Inequality of the radial pulses signifies serious disease.
b. Weak radial and normal femoral pulses are characteristic of coarctation of the aorta.
c. Pulse rate commonly increases with age.
d. Irregular pulse due to extrasystoles is accentuated during exercise.
e. Atrial fibrillation is frequently associated with a 'pulse deficit'.

Answers overleaf

6. (*a, b, d, e*)
Cardiac disease which causes inadequacy of cerebral blood flow is an important cause of transient loss of consciousness and has to be distinguished from neurological diseases (e.g. epilepsy). Syncope is not a recognized feature of coarctation of the aorta.

7. (*b*)
Pitting oedema is seen in many diseases often as the result of associated cardiac failure or hypoproteinaemia. However, the characteristic feature of lymphoedema and pretibial myxoedema is that it is non-pitting. Idiopathic portal vein thrombosis does not usually result in liver cell failure and oedema.

8. (*b, c, d, e*)
Cyanosis occurs when approximately 5 g/dl of capillary blood is desaturated and may be peripheral (due to sluggish capillary blood flow) as seen in mitral stenosis or central as in right-to-left shunts (e.g. Fallot's tetralogy, pulmonary arteriovenous shunts, and septal defects associated with severe pulmonary hypertension).

9. (*a, b, c, d*)
Epigastric pulsation is present with cardiac hypertrophy and tricuspid incompetence (due to a pulsatile liver). It is also quite common in normal thin people but reduced in coarctation of the aorta. The characteristic of an abdominal aortic aneurysm is the expansile nature of the pulsation.

10. (*e*)
Inequality of the radial pulses may signify serious disease, but it can occur in normal people who have an abnormally placed artery. Coarctation is associated with weak femoral and normal radial pulses. The pulse rate characteristically falls with age and extrasystoles tend to diminish on exercise. In atrial fibrillation the heart rate at the apex is nearly always higher than the pulse rate ('pulse deficit').

11. Which of these statements about recording the blood pressure are correct?

a. The inflatable cuff should be about 10 cm in width.
b. Auscultatory silent gap is a recognized feature of hypertension.
c. Systolic reading is usually 10 mm higher when taken by palpation rather than auscultation.
d. Diastolic reading is more accurate than the systolic.
e. An accurate reading is difficult in the presence of atrial fibrillation.

12. A collapsing pulse is a recognized feature of

a. Accelerated hypertension
b. Aortic incompetence
c. Patent ductus arteriosus
d. Hyperthyroidism
e. Congestive cardiomyopathy

13. Which of the following statements about the pulse are correct?

a. Plateau pulse is a feature of pulmonary stenosis.
b. Collapsing pulse is best felt by placing the hand around the patient's wrist with his arm held horizontally.
c. Bisferiens pulse is characteristic of combined aortic stenosis and incompetence.
d. Pulsus alternans with normal cardiac rhythm is a grave sign.
e. Jerky pulse (initial sharp rise followed by prolongation) is characteristic of tricuspid stenosis.

14. Pulsus paradoxus

a. Is where the pulse volume decreases on expiration.
b. Is characteristic of acute pericarditis.
c. Occurs in severe asthma.
d. Is associated with elevation of the jugular venous pulse during inspiration.
e. Is a recognized feature in restrictive cardiomyopathy.

Answers overleaf

11. (*a, b, e*)
The cuff should be approximately 10 cm in width as narrower ones give false readings. The systolic pressure is usually 5–10 cm lower by the palpation method; the diastolic reading is always less accurate and can only be measured by auscultation. In atrial fibrillation the stroke volume and blood pressure vary from beat to beat. If not checked by palpation, the silent gap sometimes heard in hypertensive patients can result in an erroneously low systolic reading.

12. (*b, c*)
A collapsing pulse (water hammer pulse) occurs in any condition associated with a rapid 'run-off' of blood during diastole as is present in aortic regurgitation, patent ductus arteriosus or large arteriovenous fistulae.

13. (*c, d*)
A plateau pulse (slow rising with a long summit) is characteristic of aortic stenosis; when there is also aortic incompetence a double impulse is often felt (bisferiens pulse). A collapsing pulse is best felt with the arm above the head and a jerky pulse is characteristic of obstructive cardiomyopathy. Pulsus alternans with a normal rhythm does indicate serious myocardial disease, although it may be present with a paroxysmal tachycardia without such serious implications.

14. (*c, d, e*)
Pulsus paradoxus is an accentuation of the normal fall in pulse volume on inspiration and occurs in pericardial tamponade, constrictive pericarditis, restrictive cardiomyopathies and also severe asthma. It is only present in acute pericarditis if there is a large effusion. When due to pericardial disease it is associated with an inspiratory elevation of the JVP (Kussmaul's sign).

15. Which of the following statements about the pulse are correct?

a. Vigorous arterial pulsation causing the ears to move is typical of severe aortic incompetence.
b. 'Locomotor brachial' is a sign of arteriosclerosis.
c. Capillary pulsation is recognized in hyperthyroidism.
d. 'Pistol shot' sound heard over the large arteries is characteristic of aortic stenosis.
e. A systolic murmur heard over the femoral artery is recognized in some cases of aortic regurgitation.

16. Which of the following statements about jugular veins are correct?

a. With a patient at 45° the JVP should be not more than 2 cm above the sternal angle during inspiration.
b. Jugular venous engorgement may be non-pulsatile if due to constrictive pericarditis.
c. Unilateral jugular engorgement signifies serious disease.
d. The commonest cause of a rise in venous pressure is cardiac failure.
e. Bronchial asthma is commonly associated with an elevated JVP.

17. The jugular venous pulse

a. When raised is never palpable.
b. Characteristically has two visible wave forms 'a' and 'c'.
c. May be more obvious on inspiration.
d. Shows marked 'a' waves when due to mediastinal tumours.
e. When due to congestive failure typically increases further by compression of the abdomen.

18. In normal subjects the jugular venous pulse

a. Reflects the pressure changes in the right ventricle.
b. 'a' wave is due to atrial contraction.
c. 'c' wave is due to atrial filling.
d. 'y' descent occurs after the tricuspid valve opens.
e. 'a' wave occurs after the first heart sound.

Answers overleaf

15. (*a, b, c, e*)
Vigorous arterial pulsation (Corrigan's sign) is typical of aortic incompetence, sometimes to the extent of making the ears move and the head nod. Capillary pulsation is also seen but this can occur in any cause of vasodilatation (e.g. hyperthyroidism). Murmurs over the femoral arteries are recognized in aortic regurgitation, usually a systolic murmur although occasionally a 'pistol shot' sound.

16. (*d, e*)
With a patient at 45° the JVP is at the level of the sternal angle during inspiration. Occasionally non-significant local unilateral obstruction of one jugular vein may occur which is relieved by turning the head. Apart from cardiac causes the JVP may also be elevated (principally on expiration) in conditions associated with increased intrathoracic pressure (e.g. bronchial asthma). Constrictive pericarditis, a cause of marked elevation of the JVP, may be apparently non-pulsatile because it is above the angle of the jaw.

17. (*c, e*)
The pulsation of the JVP may occasionally be palpated in the root of the neck. There are two visible waveforms ('a' and 'v') which may be more easily seen on inspiration and on compression of the abdomen. The 'a' wave is due to atrial contraction and the 'v' wave is caused by diastolic filling of the atrium. In contrast the 'c' wave due to encroachment of the tricuspid valve into the atrium during early systole is not visible. When due to mediastinal obstruction the JVP is non-pulsatile.

18. (*b, d*)
The JVP reflects right atrial pressures (*see above,* question 17). The 'a' is presystolic and thus occurs before the first heart sound, while the 'y' descent is the fall in pressure after the tricuspid valve opens.

19. Which of the following statements about the jugular venous waveforms are correct?

a. Large 'a' waves are seen in tricuspid stenosis.
b. The 'v' waves are abolished in atrial fibrillation.
c. Tall systolic waves are typical of mitral incompetence.
d. 'Cannon' waves are seen in nodal rhythm.
e. Atrial flutter is associated with intermittent 'cannon' waves.

20. In clinically significant tricuspid incompetence the JVP

a. Characteristically shows a tall systolic wave.
b. Usually does not have any 'a' waves.
c. Typically demonstrates a rapid 'y' descent.
d. Is frequently associated with 'cannon' waves.
e. May be normal in 30 per cent of cases.

21. The cardiac impulse (apex beat)

a. Is normally 10·5–12 cm from the midline.
b. Is generally in the 6th intercostal space.
c. In adult men is almost invariably within the nipple line.
d. May move up to 2 cm when lying on one side.
e. Is mainly caused by contraction of the right ventricle.

22. Lateral displacement of the apex beat is characteristic of

a. Scoliosis
b. Fibrosis of left lower lobe of the lung
c. Right-sided pleural effusion
d. Severe mitral stenosis
e. Funnel sternum (pectus excavatum)

23. Which of the following statements about a precordial thrill is correct?

a. It is more certain evidence of cardiac disease than the presence of a murmur alone.
b. In aortic stenosis the thrill is best felt in the 2nd right interspace.
c. The diastolic thrill of mitral stenosis is often easily palpable.
d. The rare combination of systolic and diastolic thrill is a recognized feature in patent ductus arteriosus.
e. It is a recognized feature in some mediastinal tumours.

Answers overleaf

19. (*a, d, e*)
The 'a' wave is very large with tricuspid stenosis and is abolished in the presence of atrial fibrillation. Tall systolic waves are caused by blood regurgitating through an incompetent tricuspid, not mitral valve. 'Cannon' waves are seen when the right atrium contracts against a closed tricuspid valve and are present in several conditions including nodal rhythms and complete heart block.

20. (*a, b, c*)
With tricuspid incompetence the 'a' wave is usually absent because of atrial fibrillation. There are large systolic waves which collapse rapidly (rapid 'y' descent).

21. (*c, d*)
The apex beat is due to contraction of the left ventricle and usually 7·5–10·5 cm (3–4 in) from the midline in the 5th intercostal space; in males this is within the nipple line. The apex beat may move up to 2 cm on change of posture.

22. (*a, b, c, e*)
Apart from cardiac disease the apex beat may be displaced laterally by skeletal deformities (scoliosis, funnel sternum), right-sided pleural effusions displacing the mediastinum or collapse of the left lung pulling the heart laterally. Mitral stenosis alone is not associated with left ventricular enlargement.

23. (All correct)
Innocent cardiac murmurs are not associated with thrills. A thrill is common in cases of aortic stenosis (usually at the 2nd right interspace) and is also often felt at the apex in cases of mitral stenosis. Thrills are not always due to valve lesions; they are felt in some vascular malformations and mediastinal tumours. A combined systolic and diastolic thrill is often felt in patent ductus arteriosus.

24. The first heart sound

a. Is associated with closure of the mitral and tricuspid valves.
b. If split, is usually associated with heart disease.
c. Is louder in patients with hyperthyroidism.
d. Is soft in mitral stenosis associated with heavy valve calcification.
e. Is best heard at the base of the heart.

25. The second heart sound

a. Is frequently split during expiration in normal individuals.
b. Reversed splitting occurs in atrial septal defect.
c. Is increased in intensity in systemic hypertension.
d. Is soft in the presence of pulmonary hypertension.
e. Exhibits fixed splitting in the presence of severe aortic stenosis.

26. The third heart sound

a. May be normal in youth.
b. Is characteristically systolic in timing.
c. Is a high-pitched sound.
d. Is a sign of severe isolated mitral stenosis.
e. Is a recognized feature of right ventricular failure.

27. The fourth heart sound

a. Is frequently heard in heart failure associated with atrial fibrillation.
b. Is a low-pitched sound.
c. Is a recognized feature of aortic stenosis.
d. Is always an abnormal sound signifying heart disease.
e. Is best heard in the aortic area.

28. An opening snap of the mitral valve

a. Is associated with mitral stenosis.
b. Indicates a calcified valve.
c. Is heard in a limited area at the left sternal edge.
d. Is typically of longer duration than a third sound.
e. Is closer to the second heart sound in severe stenosis.

Answers overleaf

24. (*a, c, d*)
The first heart sound, which is due to closure of the mitral and tricuspid valves in health, is often narrowly split and best heard at the apex of the heart. It is louder with increased activity of the heart (e.g. hyperthyroidism) and mitral stenosis, provided the valve is not heavily calcified.

25. (*c*)
Normal splitting of the second heart sound occurs on inspiration due to increased venous return to the heart. Fixed splitting is associated with atrial septal defect and reversed splitting (narrowing of the sound on inspiration) with left bundle-branch block. The aortic second sound is loud with systemic hypertension and the pulmonary second sound with pulmonary arterial hypertension.

26. (*a, e*)
The third heart sound is low pitched, diastolic in timing and may be heard in some normal young people. It most frequently occurs in conditions causing left ventricular dysfunction (this is not the case with isolated mitral stenosis). Occasionally, a third heart sound originates from the right ventricle.

27. (*b, c, d*)
The fourth heart sound occurs when atrial contraction forces blood into either the right or left ventricle when the end-diastolic pressure is high (e.g. in heart failure or aortic stenosis). Thus the sound does not occur in the presence of atrial fibrillation. It is a low-pitched sound and is best heard parasternally or in the epigastrium.

28. (*a, e*)
An opening snap is a sign of mitral stenosis but is only present with a mobile valve. Unlike the third heart sound it is short and sharp. It is frequently heard widely over the precordium and the closer it occurs to the second sound the tighter the valve stenosis.

29. Which of the following statements about clicks are correct?

a. Ejection clicks occur immediately after the first heart sound.
b. Mid-systolic clicks may be associated with mitral stenosis.
c. Pulmonary valve stenosis is a recognized cause of an ejection click.
d. Valve calcification results in louder clicks.
e. Ejection clicks are more common in conditions associated with delayed opening of the semilunar valves.

30. Pericardial friction

a. Is nearly always absent in the presence of a significant pericardial effusion.
b. Is always a systolic scratchy sound.
c. Is characteristically accentuated in certain positions.
d. Is typically painless.
e. Is always widely distributed over the precordium.

31. Which of the following statements about murmurs are correct?

a. Murmurs should be timed by feeling the radial pulse.
b. Presystolic murmurs immediately precede the first heart sound.
c. There is a relationship between the loudness of a murmur and the haemodynamic severity of the cardiac lesion.
d. Aortic systolic murmurs characteristically vary with respiration.
e. Aortic diastolic murmur is best heard in the left lateral position.

32. Which of the following are true of innocent cardiac murmurs?

a. Are always systolic in timing.
b. Nearly always occur in the aortic area.
c. Are typically louder on exercise.
d. Are occasionally associated with a fourth heart sound.
e. Are most often 'ejection' in type (mid-systolic).

Answers overleaf

29. (*a, c, e*)
Ejection clicks occur immediately after the first heart sound and are due to the sudden opening of the semilunar valves in conditions associated with delayed valve opening (e.g. aortic or pulmonary stenosis). Calcification diminishes or abolishes an ejection click. The mid-systolic click is associated with mitral valve prolapse not stenosis.

30. (*c*)
Pericardial friction may occur during any part of the cardiac cycle, is usually associated with pain and can be localized or generalized in distribution. In the presence of effusion pericardial friction is usually heard.

31. (*b*)
Because of the delay involved murmurs cannot be timed from the radial pulse; timing must always be from the carotid pulse or cardiac impulse. Presystolic murmurs immediately precede the first heart sound. Although there is no relationship between the loudness of a murmur and the haemodynamic disturbance, loud murmurs are nearly always due to organic disease. It is pulmonary systolic murmurs which characteristically vary with respiration. Aortic diastolic murmurs are heard in expiration at the left sternal edge, with the patient leaning forwards.

32. (*a, c, e*)
Innocent murmurs which are nearly always mid-systolic in timing are most commonly heard in the pulmonary area and like many other murmurs are louder on exercise. A fourth heart sound is always pathological.

33. A pansystolic murmur heard at the apex of the heart may be due to

a. Pulmonary stenosis
b. Ventricular septal defect
c. Tricuspid regurgitation
d. Papillary muscle dysfunction
e. Atrial septal defect

34. Mitral valve prolapse

a. Is associated with an early systolic click.
b. Is associated with a late systolic murmur.
c. May be best heard in the parasternal area.
d. Can easily be confused with the murmur of aortic stenosis.
e. In most cases results in cardiac failure.

35. Mitral diastolic murmur

a. Only occurs with an abnormal valve.
b. Is characteristically high pitched.
c. Is typically localized to the apex.
d. May be accentuated in the right lateral position.
e. Is softer after exercise.

36. Aortic systolic murmurs are a recognized feature of

a. Anaemias
b. Calcification of the aortic root
c. Hypertrophic cardiomyopathy
d. Systemic hypertension
e. Dilatation of the aorta

37. The murmur of aortic stenosis typically

a. Is widely distributed over the precordium.
b. Is mid-diastolic in timing.
c. Is associated with a palpable thrill.
d. Radiates to the axillae.
e. Is associated with an early systolic click.

Answers overleaf

33. (*b, c, d*)
An apical pansystolic murmur is due to mitral regurgitation, ventricular septal defect or tricuspid regurgitation (i.e. those conditions in which there is a gradient across the diseased valve or septum throughout systole). Atrial septal defects are associated with murmurs from the pulmonary valve.

34. (*b, c, d*)
The click of mitral prolapse is mid-systolic and associated with a late systolic murmur, which may be best heard parasternally and hence confused with aortic stenosis. In many cases there is no haemodynamic disturbance.

35. (*c*)
Mitral diastolic murmurs may rarely be heard with a normal valve due to increased blood flow in left-to-right shunts and aortic regurgitation ('Austin Flint murmur'). Such murmurs are characteristically low pitched and rumbling, accentuated in the left lateral position and on exercise and typically localized to the apex of the heart.

36. (*a, b, c, e*)
Aortic systolic murmurs are very common and may not be associated with valve disease. Calcification of the aortic root is a common cause, particularly in the elderly, and frequently does not result in clinically significant stenosis. Hypertrophic cardiomyopathy is a rare cause of subvalvular aortic and pulmonary stenosis. Systemic hypertension alone is not a cause of aortic systolic murmurs.

37. (*a, c, e*)
Aortic stenosis is characterized by a widely distributed rough mid-systolic murmur which typically radiates to the carotid arteries and is often associated with a palpable thrill. It may be preceded by an early systolic click.

38. The murmur of aortic regurgitation

a. Is usually best heard at the left sternal edge.
b. Is high pitched.
c. Occurs in late diastole.
d. Is accentuated with the patient leaning forwards and holding his breath in expiration.
e. Radiates to the neck.

39. Which of the following statements about murmurs in the pulmonary area are correct?

a. In the majority of cases systolic murmurs are benign.
b. With pulmonary stenosis there is a delay in the pulmonary second sound.
c. They may be indistinguishable from aortic valve lesions.
d. Pulmonary incompetent murmur radiates to the back.
e. A Graham Steell murmur arises from the pulmonary valve.

40. Which of the following statements about tricuspid valve disease are correct?

a. In nearly every case tricuspid stenosis is due to rheumatic heart disease.
b. Tricuspid stenosis is associated with large flicking 'a' waves in the JVP.
c. If severe, tricuspid incompetence is associated with presystolic pulsation of the liver.
d. Tricuspid murmurs are made louder on inspiration.
e. Tricuspid incompetence is associated with the 'bruit de diable'.

41. Which of the following statements about the electrocardiograph are correct?

a. The usual standardization is 1 cm for 1 mV.
b. P waves are absent in atrial fibrillation.
c. The P–R interval is reduced in digitalis poisoning.
d. The axis deviation of the heart is best shown in leads V1 and V3.
e. Negative T waves in leads II and III may occur temporarily with fevers.

Answers overleaf

38. (*a, b, d*)
Aortic regurgitation produces a high-pitched, soft, early diastolic murmur best heard at the left sternal edge with the patient leaning forwards and holding his breath in expiration. It may be heard in the axillae but not in the neck.

39. (*a, b, c, e*)
Murmurs in the pulmonary area are most commonly benign. However, when due to valve disease they are frequently indistinguishable from aortic valve disease. Pulmonary stenosis is associated with a delay of the pulmonary second sound. The so-called Graham Steell murmur is associated with dilatation of the pulmonary artery as occurs with severe mitral valve disease or Eisenmenger's reaction.

40. (*a, b, d*)
Tricuspid stenosis is nearly always rheumatic in nature and occurs in about 10 per cent of cases of rheumatic heart disease. Tricuspid stenosis is associated with large 'a' waves in the JVP and presystolic pulsation of the liver. In tricuspid incompetence there is a large systolic wave in the JVP and the liver exhibits systolic pulsation. Tricuspid murmurs are louder on inspiration. *Bruit de diable* is a venous hum heard over the neck in profound anaemias.

41. (*a, b, e*)
The normal standardization for an ECG is 1 cm for 1 mV. The P wave due to atrial contraction is absent in atrial fibrillation and P–R interval increased in digitalis poisoning. The easiest way to decide the electrical axis of the heart is to look at the R waves in standard leads I and III. Negative T waves in the inferior leads (II, III and aVF) may occur with fevers.

42. The following are recognized causes of pericarditis:

a. Rheumatic fever
b. Rheumatoid arthritis
c. Tuberculosis
d. Uraemia
e. Pneumonia

43. Pericardial tamponade is typically associated with the following clinical features:

a. Third heart sound
b. Parasternal impulse
c. Inspiratory rise in the JVP
d. Pulsus alternans
e. Pericardial friction rub

44. Constrictive pericarditis is generally associated with

a. Previous tuberculous infection
b. Ascites
c. Loud first heart sound
d. Globular cardiac shadow on the chest X-ray
e. Calcification of the pericardium

45. Myocardial infarction is associated with the following complications:

a. Cerebrovasular accident
b. Mitral regurgitation
c. Complete heart block
d. Left ventricular aneurysm
e. Pericarditis

46. The following are typical features of mitral stenosis:

a. Accentuated first heart sound
b. Rumbling systolic murmur
c. Bifid P waves on the ECG
d. Peripheral cyanosis
e. Left ventricular enlargement on the chest radiograph

Answers overleaf

42. (All correct)
These are some of the many causes of pericardial effusions.

43. (*a, c, e*)
If a pericardial effusion is large enough, it restricts cardiac output (cardiac tamponade). This situation is associated with pulsus paradoxus, an inspiratory rise in the JVP (Kussmaul's sign), a feeble cardiac impulse, a third heart sound and in most cases pericardial friction.

44. (*a, b, e*)
Constrictive pericarditis due to contraction of the pericardium also restricts the cardiac output and thus produces similar physical signs to pericardial tamponade. Ascites is relatively common as is pericardial calcification. Unlike pericardial effusion the heart shadow on the chest X-ray is not usually globular.

45. (All correct)
Myocardial infarction is associated with many complications. Cerebrovascular accident may be caused by a mural embolism, mitral regurgitation by papillary muscle dysfunction or rupture of a chordae tendineae; pericarditis is secondary to transmural infarction or the post-myocardial infarction syndrome. Left ventricular aneurysm occurs in 10–20 per cent of patients and is due to dilatation of scar tissue after infarction.

46. (*a, c, d*)
The clinical signs associated with mitral stenosis include peripheral cyanosis, loud first heart sound, opening snap and rumbling diastolic murmur localized to the apex. If the heart is in sinus rhythm the P waves on the ECG are bifid (P mitrale). In pure mitral stenosis the left ventricle is small.

47. Mitral incompetence

a. Is invariably associated with a pansystolic murmur.
b. Is a recognized complication of heart failure.
c. Due to ruptured chordae tendineae is typically asymptomatic.
d. If severe, is associated with a tapping apex beat.
e. In most cases is associated with a third heart sound.

48. Which of the following statements about aortic incompetence are correct?

a. Capillary pulsation is diagnostic.
b. Pulmonary hypertension is a usual feature.
c. An Austin Flint murmur is a recognized feature.
d. Aortic incompetence is associated with Marfan's syndrome.
e. The cardiac rhythm is typically atrial fibrillation.

49. Advanced aortic stenosis is characterized by

a. Collapsing pulse
b. Fourth heart sound
c. Localized rough mid-systolic murmur
d. Angina pectoris
e. Syncope

50. The following are suggestive of bacterial endocarditis:

a. Increasing valve stenosis
b. Petechiae in the skin
c. Splenomegaly
d. Heberden's nodes
e. Anaemia

51. The following are typical manifestations of an atrial septal defect:

a. Fixed splitting of the second heart sound
b. Systolic murmur due to the left-to-right shunt
c. Mid-diastolic murmur in the tricuspid area
d. Left-bundle branch block
e. Pulsus paradoxus

Answers overleaf

47. (*b, e*)
Mitral incompetence can be due to many different causes (e.g. rheumatic heart disease, heart failure, myocardial infarction, bacterial endocarditis). The murmur is usually pansystolic, but in the case of papillary muscle dysfunction it may be late systolic in timing. In nearly every case there is a third heart sound and the first sound is soft, hence a tapping apex beat does not occur. Ruptured chordae tendineae result in severe life-threatening heart failure.

48. (*c, d*)
Although capillary pulsation is a feature of aortic incompetence, it occurs with any cause of high cardiac output. Pulmonary hypertension is not a feature and the heart is usually in sinus rhythm. An Austin Flint murmur is a feature of severe aortic incompetence (*see* Question 35).

49. (*b, d, e*)
The main characteristics of aortic stenosis are a plateau pulse and widespread rough mid-systolic murmur. Angina pectoris and syncopal attacks are common and may be due to poor perfusion of the coronary arteries. A fourth heart sound is very common.

50. (*b, c, e*)
Bacterial endocarditis destroys cardiac valves and is therefore associated with valve incompetence. Petechiae, finger clubbing, Osler's nodes, splenomegaly and anaemia are typical features of the condition. Heberden's nodes are caused by osteoarthritis.

51. (*a, c*)
In atrial septal defect the left-to-right shunt is silent. However, increased blood flow often produces a mid-diastolic murmur in the tricuspid area and a mid-systolic murmur in the pulmonary area. There is fixed splitting of the second heart sound and the ECG usually shows right-bundle branch block.

52. A large asymptomatic ventricular septal defect is generally associated with

a. Mid-diastolic murmur at the apex
b. Systemic hypertension
c. Pansystolic murmur in the left parasternal region
d. Complete heart block
e. Small pulmonary artery on the chest radiograph

53. Typical clinical accompaniments of patent ductus arteriosus are

a. Right ventricular enlargement
b. Small peripheral pulse pressure
c. Continuous murmur (systolic and diastolic)
d. Right-bundle branch block on the ECG
e. High-arched palate

54. Fallot's tetralogy is associated with

a. Mid-systolic murmur in the second left interspace
b. Heaving apex beat
c. Central cyanosis
d. Left-bundle branch block
e. Finger clubbing

55. The following are recognized features of coarctation of the aorta:

a. Late systolic murmur heard over the scapula
b. Mental retardation
c. Fractures of the ribs
d. Hypertensive changes in the optic fundi
e. Collapsing pulse

56. Extrasystoles

a. Are beats of bigger volume than normal.
b. When coupled (occurring every second beat), usually signify digoxin toxicity.
c. Increase on exercise.
d. Typically produce an irregularly irregular pulse.
e. In most cases are associated with myocardial disease.

Answers overleaf

52. (*a, c*)
Unlike an atrial defect the blood flow through a ventricular septal defect usually produces a pansystolic murmur in the parasternal area. Increased flow across the mitral valve may result in an apical mid-diastolic murmur, and the large volume of blood passing through the lungs results in the pulmonary artery being more prominent than normal.

53. (*c*)
The continuous shunting of blood from aorta to pulmonary artery may result in left ventricular hypertrophy and invariably causes a continuous murmur (machinery murmur). The pulse pressure is high and is associated with capillary pulsation. High-arched palate and right-bundle branch block are not features of this condition.

54. (*a, b, c, e*)
Fallot's tetralogy is associated with pulmonary stenosis and a ventricular septal defect. There is usually a right-to-left shunt (and therefore cyanosis and finger clubbing) because of the resistance imposed by the pulmonary stenosis. Right ventricular hypertrophy is invariably present, the second heart sound is single and there is nearly always a systolic murmur heard in the second interspace.

55. (*a, d*)
Coarctation of the aorta results in extensive collateral vessels around the scapulae (producing a late systolic murmur). Enlargement of the intercostal arteries results in rib notching (not fractures). Hypertension above the coarctation results in characteristic changes in the optic fundi. Mental retardation and a collapsing pulse are not features.

56. (*b*)
The extrasystolic beat is small in volume followed by a large volume sinus beat. Atrial fibrillation typically produces an irregularly irregular pulse; however, sometimes it can be difficult to distinguish between atrial fibrillation and multiple ectopic beats. Coupled beats are usually a sign of digoxin toxicity. In most cases ectopic beats decrease on exercise and do not signify underlying heart disease.

57. Which of the following statements about atrial fibrillation are correct?

a. Stroke volume of the left ventricle varies from beat to beat.
b. The atrial rate is typically over 400 contractions per min.
c. The pulse rate is often higher than the heart rate at the apex.
d. The 'a' wave in the JVP becomes more prominent.
e. It encourages thrombus formation in the atria.

58. Atrial fibrillation is a recognized complication of

a. Mitral stenosis
b. Carcinoma of the bronchus
c. Thyrotoxicosis
d. Ischaemic heart disease
e. Acute chest infections

59. The following are characteristic features of atrial flutter:

a. Irregular heart beat
b. Cannon waves in the JVP
c. Sudden doubling of the heart rate
d. Slowing with carotid sinus massage
e. Pulsus alternans

60. Recognized features of paroxysmal atrial tachycardia include

a. Heart rate of 140–160 beats/min.
b. Angina pectoris
c. Pulsus paradoxus
d. Syncope
e. Polyuria

61. Sinus bradycardia is a recognized feature

a. With increased intercranial pressure
b. Following influenza
c. In athletes
d. In myxoedema
e. With jaundice

Answers overleaf

57. (*a, b, e*)
The irregularity of ventricular beats in atrial fibrillation results in varying stroke volume some of the beats being of such low volume that the pulse rate is often apparently slower than the apex rate. The atrial rate varies from 400 to 600 contractions per min. The lack of effective atrial emptying results in stasis of blood particularly in the atrial appendage and thrombus formation. The 'a' wave in the JVP is due to atrial contraction and is therefore absent in the presence of atrial fibrillation.

58. (All correct)
All these conditions (and several more besides) predispose to atrial fibrillation.

59. (*b, c, d*)
In atrial flutter there is a regular atrioventricular block, and so the tachycardia is regular but may suddenly double or halve in rate (the latter is especially liable to occur with carotid sinus massage). Cannon waves in the JVP occur when the right atrium contracts against a closed tricuspid valve.

60. (*a, b, d, e*)
Paroxysmal atrial tachycardia is commonly at a rate of 140–160 beats/min and as with any tachycardia may precipitate angina pectoris. Syncope sometimes occurs particularly at the onset of the arrhythmia. Polyuria is a common symptom.

61. (All correct)
Sinus bradycardia applies to heart rates below 60 beats/min and occurs in some healthy elderly people and in trained athletes. It can also occur after viral illnesses, with myxoedema, raised intracranial pressure and jaundice.

62. Characteristic features of complete heart block include

a. Pulse rate of 60 beats/min
b. Frequent syncopal attacks
c. Varying intensity of the first heart sound
d. Tall V waves in the JVP
e. Dicrotic pulse

63. Left ventricular failure is associated with

a. Raised left atrial pressure
b. Pleural effusions
c. Frothy sputum
d. Third and fourth heart sounds
e. Ascites

64. The following are recognized clinical features of right ventricular failure:

a. Impaired renal function
b. Right hypochondrial pain
c. Splenomegaly
d. Haemoptysis
e. Non-pitting ankle oedema

65. Causes of congestive cardiac failure include

a. Chronic obstructive bronchitis
b. Multiple pulmonary embolism
c. Chronic alcoholism
d. Ischaemic heart disease
e. Hyperthyroidism

66. In obliterative arterial disease of the legs

a. Pain is typically eased by exercise.
b. There is loss of hair on the affected limb.
c. If the legs are elevated then lowered, the colour returns more quickly on the affected side.
d. A bruit is most commonly heard over the tibial pulses.
e. Parasthesia is a typical symptom.

Answers overleaf

62. (*b, c*)
The heart rate in complete heart block is usually between 20 and 50 beats/min and there is a tendency for periods of ventricular standstill resulting in syncope (Stokes–Adams attacks). Cannon waves (not tall V waves) are seen in the JVP and the first heart sound varies in intensity. Dicrotic pulse occurs when low stroke output is associated with peripheral vasodilatation and not with complete heart block.

63. (*a, c, d*)
When the left ventricle fails, then the left atrial pressure and pulmonary venous pressure increases. If this is of sufficient degree, pulmonary oedema will occur. Orthopnoea is an early symptom of pulmonary oedema and frothy blood-tinged sputum a late manifestation. Third and fourth heart sounds are often noted but ascites and pleural effusions will only be present if there is right heart failure.

64. (*a, b*)
Right ventricular failure is typically associated with elevation of the JVP, enlarged liver often causing right hypochondrial pain, pitting oedema of the ankles and ascites. Haemoptysis and splenomegaly are not usual findings.

65. (All correct)
Congestive cardiac failure is most commonly caused by ischaemic heart disease, hypertension or chronic bronchitis. Rarer causes are multiple pulmonary emboli, hyperthyroidism (in the elderly this may be the first manifestation of an overactive thyroid) and alcoholism.

66. (*b, e*)
Claudication, the pain caused by arterial insufficiency, is typically made worse by exercise. There is often loss of hair on the affected limb and parasthesia may also occur. A bruit, if present, is heard over the large vessels, not the tibial pulses. On elevating and then lowering the leg the colour returns more slowly to the affected limb.

67. Systemic hypertension

a. Is typically associated with headaches.
b. Is a complication of Addison's disease.
c. Is associated with retinal haemorrhages.
d. Is a recognized cause of congestive cardiac failure.
e. Is a characteristic finding in acute glomerular nephritis.

68. Raynaud phenomenon

a. Typically occurs in young men.
b. Is associated with the use of pneumatic drills.
c. Is a recognized feature of scleroderma.
d. Is precipitated by cold.
e. Is complicated by painful ulcers.

69. Cutaneous vasculitis is a feature of

a. Polyarteritis nodosa
b. Polymyalgia rheumatica (painful stiffness of the proximal limb muscles)
c. Systemic sclerosis
d. Rheumatoid disease
e. Neurofibromatosis

70. Which of the following statements about venous thrombosis are correct?

a. Thrombophlebitis migrans is a complication of malignant disease.
b. Deep vein thrombosis is invariably associated with swelling of the leg.
c. Low-grade fever is a typical feature of deep vein thrombosis.
d. The oral contraceptive predisposes to varicose veins.
e. Varicose ulcers are typically found on the lateral aspect of the lower leg.

Answers overleaf

67. (*c, d, e*)
Hypertension is usually asymptomatic and discovered at routine medical examinations. In the majority of cases no underlying cause is found; however, a few patients will be suffering from renal disease, endocrine disease (Cushing's syndrome or phaeochromocytoma) or coarctation of the aorta. Addison's disease results in hypotension. Haemorrhages and papilloedema are seen in the optic fundi of severe cases.

68. (*b, c, d, e*)
Raynaud phenomenon is typically seen in young women, a proportion of whom have scleroderma. One rare cause in men is the prolonged use of pneumatic drills. This condition is precipitated by cold and occasionally results in painful ulcers on the fingers.

69. (*a, b, c, d*)
Cutaneous vasculitis is an uncommon feature of the collagen diseases, but not of neurofibromatosis or polymyalgia rheumatica.

70. (*a, b, c*)
Thrombophlebitis migrans is usually associated with underlying malignancy (particularly carcinoma of the pancreas). With deep vein thrombosis low-grade pyrexia is common but swelling of the leg is not always present. Venous ulcers are typically found on the medial aspect of the lower leg.

1. A man aged 65 with good previous health woke up in the early hours of the morning with intense dyspnoea and a cough productive of thin frothy sputum. He had to sit out of bed for the remainder of the night.
   a. What is the probable cause of this attack?
   b. List four abnormal physical signs which might be present.

2. A previously fit 70-year-old man developed sudden very severe retrosternal chest pain. He was found to have a pulse rate of 45 beats/min and blood pressure of 100/70 mm. He then had two transient convulsions.
   a. What is the diagnosis and what complication has he developed?
   b. Why did he have convulsions?
   c. Name one associated physical sign in the jugular veins.
   d. What special treatment must be considered?

3. A 50-year-old woman presented with sudden onset of palpitations and mild dyspnoea. Her pulse was irregular at 140 beats/min.
   a. What is the likely arrythmia?
   b. Gives three causes for this arrythmia.

4. A 60-year-old man complained of tiredness and dyspnoea. His blood pressure was 90/70, pulse was low volume and disappeared on inspiration, heart sounds were soft and a systolic murmur heard over the precordium was also reported.
   a. What is the diagnosis?
   b. Give two causes of this condition.
   c. What is the likely explanation of the murmur?
   d. Give two other characteristic physical signs.

5. A 69-year-old woman who had suffered from chorea as a child and had an operation on her heart 20 years ago presented in congestive cardiac failure. She had a left thoracotomy scar, fast irregular pulse, loud first heart sound and a long mid-diastolic murmur. There was a pansystolic murmur best heard at the left sternal edge and loudest on inspiration. Large systolic waves were seen in the jugular veins.
   a. Name two likely valve lesions.
   b. What was the operation 20 years ago?
   c. List three other physical signs which might be present.

Answers overleaf

1. *a*. Left ventricular failure
b. (i) Basal inspiratory crackles
(ii) Systemic hypertension
(iii) Thrusting left ventricular impulse
(iv) Third or fourth heart sound
(v) Atrial fibrillation
(vi) Aortic or mitral systolic murmurs

2. *a*. Myocardial infarction and complete heart block
b. Cerebral anoxia due to a period of asystole
c. Cannon waves
d. Cardiac pacemaker

3. *a*. Atrial fibrillation
b. (i) Ischaemic heart disease
(ii) Thyrotoxicosis
(iii) Mitral stenosis

4. *a*. Pericardial effusion with tamponade
b. (i) Systemic lupus erythematosus
(ii) Pneumococcal pericarditis
c. Pericardial friction rub
d. (i) High jugular venous pressure with further elevation on inspiration (Kussmaul's sign)
(ii) Systolic added sound, 'pericardial knock'

5. *a*. (i) Mitral stenosis
(ii) Tricuspid incompetence
b. Closed mitral valvotomy
c. (i) Right ventricular impulse
(ii) Opening snap
(iii) Systolic pulsation of the liver

Arrange the following associations into their correct pairs:

1. *A*. Cheyne–Stokes breathing
B. Hepatomegaly
C. Syncope
D. Non-pitting leg oedema
E. Expansile epigastric pulsation

a. Abdominal aortic aneurysm
b. Severe left-heart failure
c. Right-heart failure
d. Aortic stenosis
e. Myxoedema

2. *A*. Pulsus paradoxus
B. Jerky pulse
C. Collapsing pulse
D. Plateau pulse
E. Bisferiens pulse

a. Combined aortic incompetence and stenosis
b. Aortic incompetence
c. Obstructive cardiomyopathy
d. Pericardial tamponade
e. Aortic stenosis

3. *A*. Cyanosis
B. 'Pulse deficit'
C. Capillary pulsation
D. 'Locomotor brachial'
E. Small pulse pressure

a. Aortic incompetence
b. Aortic stenosis
c. Atrial fibrillation
d. Pulmonary arteriovenous shunt
e. Arteriosclerosis

4. *A*. Large A waves in jugular veins
B. Cannon waves in jugular veins
C. Absent A waves in jugular veins
D. Lateral displacement of apex beat
E. Inspiratory rise in jugular veins

a. Pericardial tamponade
b. Funnel chest
c. Complete heart block
d. Atrial fibrillation
e. Tricuspid stenosis

5. *A*. Loud first heart sound
B. Reversed splitting of second heart sound
C. Loud aortic second sound
D. Fixed splitting of second heart sound
E. Mid-diastolic click

a. Mitral valve prolapse
b. Left-bundle branch block
c. Mitral stenosis
d. Hypertension
e. Atrial septal defect

Answers overleaf

1. *A*......*b*
B......*c*
C......*d*
D......*e*
E......*a*

2. *A*......*d*
B......*c*
C......*b*
D......*e*
E......*a*

3. *A*......*d*
B......*c*
C......*a*
D......*e*
E......*b*

4. *A*......*e*
B......*c*
C......*d*
D......*b*
E......*a*

5. *A*......*c*
B......*b*
C......*d*
D......*e*
E......*a*

6. *A*. Pericardial friction
B. Diastolic murmur (left sternal edge)
C. Mitral diastolic murmur
D. Mid-systolic murmur (2nd interspace)
E. Presystolic liver pulsation

a. Aortic stenosis
b. Mitral stenosis
c. Tricuspid incompetence
d. Myocardial infarction
e. Aortic incompetence

7. *A*. Prolonged PR interval on ECG
B. Deep Q waves
C. Transient ST segment depression
D. Bifid P waves
E. Tall P waves

a. Mitral stenosis
b. Cor pulmonale
c. Effort angina
d. Digoxin toxicity
e. Myocardial infarction

8. *A*. Tapping apex beat
B. Pericardial calcification
C. Venous hum in neck
D. Splenomegaly
E. Continuous murmur

a. Bacterial endocarditis
b. Patent ductus arteriosus
c. Mitral stenosis
d. Tuberculosis
e. Anaemia

9. *A*. Finger clubbing
B. Rib notching
C. Variable pulse pressure
D. Cannon waves
E. Livido reticularis

a. Coarctation of the aorta
b. Atrial flutter
c. Systemic lupus erythematosus
d. Fallot's tetralogy
e. Atrial fibrillation

10. *A*. Ascites (transudate)
B. Raynaud phenomenon
C. Thrombophlebitis migrans
D. Dissecting aortic aneurysm
E. *Bruit de diable*

a. Scleroderma
b. Tricuspid incompetence
c. Severe anaemia
d. Malignancy
e. Marfan's syndrome

Answers overleaf

6. *A......d*
B......e
C......b
D......a
E......c

7. *A......d*
B......e
C......c
D......a
E......b

8. *A......c*
B......d
C......e
D......a
E......b

9. *A......d*
B......a
C......e
D......b
E......c

10. *A......b*
B......a
C......d
D......e
E......c

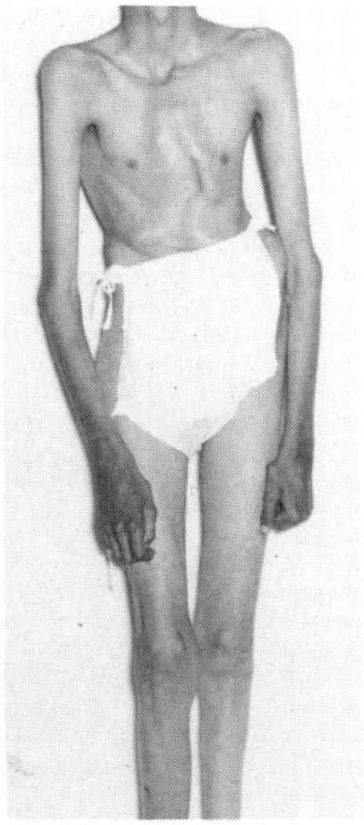

Fig. 7.1

a. Name the syndrome shown here.

b. List three non-skeletal signs which might be found.

Answers overleaf

Fig. 7.1

a. Marfan's syndrome

b. Dislocated lens ('shimmering' of iris on rapid eye movement); cardiac murmurs (aortic incompetence especially); signs of spontaneous pneumothorax

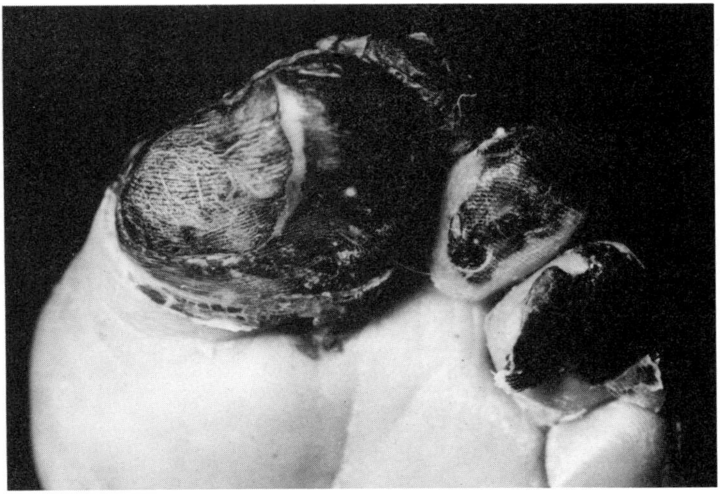

Fig. 7.2
a. What is this condition?
b. Give three possible causes.

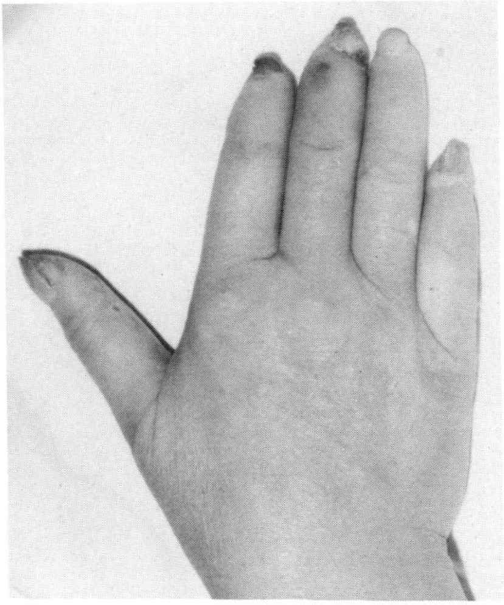

Fig. 7.3
a. Describe the abnormalities shown.
b. List three internal organs which might be affected in this patient.

Answers overleaf

Fig. 7.2
a. Gangrene
b. Atheroma; diabetes; frost-bite

Fig. 7.3
a. Necrosis of terminal phalanges with shrinkage and blackening of overlying nails; skin of fingers smooth with loss of normal wrinkles (fifth finger especially); scleroderma
b. Oesophagus; lungs; heart; small bowel (all can be affected in systemic sclerosis)

The Haemopoietic System

(Refer to Chapter 8 in *Symptoms and Signs in Clinical Medicine*, 11th edition, p. 295.)

1. Typical features of severe anaemia include

a. Anorexia
b. Dizziness
c. Dyspnoea
d. Effort angina
e. Retinal haemorrhages

2. Generalized lymphadenopathy is typical of

a. Glandular fever (infectious mononucleosis)
b. Carcinoma of the bronchus
c. Tuberculous lymphadenopathy
d. Chronic lymphatic leukaemia
e. Non-Hodgkin's lymphoma

3. Which of the following statements about lymph nodes are correct?

a. Nodes due to carcinoma are usually painful.
b. Nodes are adherent to underlying tissues in lymphoma.
c. Cervical lymphadenopathy in children is a grave sign.
d. In lymphoma the nodes are usually of a rubbery consistency.
e. Stony hard and irregular nodes are typically due to carcinoma.

4. The following are characteristics of an enlarged spleen:

a. It moves up on inspiration.
b. If grossly enlarged, it is possible to get above the swelling.
c. Dullness to percussion is typically over the 9th to 11th ribs.
d. A palpable notch is pathognomonic.
e. It lies parallel to the rib margin.

5. Causes of massive enlargement of the spleen include

a. Megaloblastic anaemia
b. Myelofibrosis
c. Miliary tuberculosis
d. Kala-azar
e. Malaria

Answers overleaf

1. (All correct)
Most symptoms due to anaemia result from the reduced oxygen-carrying capacity of the blood (*a, b, c, d*). Retinal haemorrhages may be present in severe anaemia of any aetiology.

2. (*a, d, e*)
Generalized enlargement of the lymphatic glands occurs most commonly with malignancy of the lymphatic system or with certain infections (e.g. glandular fever). Carinoma of the bronchus and tuberculosis are frequently associated with lymphadenopathy but typically this only involves certain groups of glands.

3. (*d, e*)
Painful nodes are usually infected while those infiltrated with malignant cells are generally painless. Lymphoma glands usually have a rubbery consistency while carcinomatous glands are very hard and frequently fixed to deep structures. Cervical lymphadenopathy is very common in childhood and only rarely signifies malignant disease.

4. (*c, d, e*)
The spleen, if felt with the patient recumbent, lies parallel to the lower left rib margin. It moves down on inspiration and it is never possible to get above the swelling. A notch is only occasionally felt but is pathognomonic. The percussion note is dull over the 9th to 11th ribs.

5. (*b, d, e*)
These are all causes of splenomegaly. However, only myelofibrosis, malaria and kala-azar cause massive splenic enlargement.

6. Recognized causes of optic atrophy in an anaemic patient include

a. Vitamin B_{12} deficiency
b. Massive haemorrhage
c. Vitamin C deficiency
d. Mild chronic blood loss
e. Hypothyroidism

7. Which of the following statements concerning mouth abnormalities are correct?

a. Depapillated tongue is associated with iron deficiency.
b. Gum hypertrophy is a recognized complication of acute leukaemia.
c. Lymphatic leukaemic deposits may cause gross tonsillar enlargement.
d. Mouth ulceration is a recognized manifestation of vitamin B_{12} deficiency.
e. Sponginess of the gums is associated with vitamin C deficiency.

8. Haemoglobin

a. Estimation is performed spectrophotometrically.
b. Concentration of 10 g/dl is normal for young women.
c. Mean corpuscular concentration (MCHC) is derived from the haemoglobin concentration and packed-cell volume.
d. MCHC is normal in macrocytic anaemias.
e. Packed-cell volume (PCV) is low in polycythaemia.

9. Which of the following statements about red-cell morphology are correct?

a. Poikilocytosis is typically seen in myelofibrosis.
b. Target cells are associated with polycythaemia.
c. Basophilic stippling is characteristic of sickle-cell anaemia.
d. Howell–Jolly bodies are seen after splenectomy.
e. Rouleaux formation is typically seen in multiple myeloma.

Answers overleaf

6. (*a, b*)
Optic atrophy is a well-recognized sequela of vitamin B_{12} deficiency. Retinal haemorrhages secondary to severe blood loss very occasionally lead to optic atrophy.

7. (All correct)
The tongue in severe iron deficiency is depapillated, while with vitamin B_{12} and folate deficiency it is red and raw. Both leukaemia and prolonged phenytoin administration cause gum hypertrophy. Mouth ulceration is typical of leukaemia, agranulocytosis and vitamin B_{12} deficiency.

8. (*a, c, d*)
Haemoglobin concentration is estimated spectrophotometrically after converting it to cyanmethaemoglobin. The lower normal range for young women is 11·5 g/100 ml. The mean corpuscular haemoglobin concentration derived by dividing the haemoglobin concentration by the packed-cell volume (×100) is low in iron deficiency but normal in megaloblastic anaemia. The PCV is always high in polycythaemia.

9. (*a, d, e*)
Variation in the shape of red cells (poikilocytosis) is characteristic of myelofibrosis and megaloblastic anaemias. Target cells are generally seen with hypochromic anaemia, haemoglobinopathies, liver disease and after splenectomy. Basophilic stippling is associated with toxic states particularly lead poisoning. Howell–Jolly bodies (nuclear remnants) are typical of post-splenectomy states and hyposplenism (as may also be associated with coeliac disease).

10. Increased numbers of white cells in the peripheral blood are associated with

a. Pregnancy
b. Myocardial infarction
c. Felty's syndrome
d. Megaloblastic anaemia
e. Severe exercise

11. Features of agranulocytosis include

a. Dysphagia
b. Delayed wound healing
c. Generalized lymphadenitis
d. Severe lassitude
e. Bronchospasm

12. Thrombocythaemia is a recognized feature of

a. Mycoplasma infections
b. Polycythaemia
c. Acute haemorrhage
d. Corticosteroid therapy
e. Chronic myeloid leukaemia

13. A large loss of blood is associated with

a. Immediate fall in haemoglobin concentration
b. Polychromatic red cells
c. Rise in platelet count
d. Fall in packed-cell volume
e. Leucocytosis

14. The following are features of iron deficiency:

a. Dysphagia
b. Grey coloration of the skin
c. Koilonychia
d. Aphthous ulceration
e. Peripheral neuropathy

Answers overleaf

10. (*a, b, e*)
Leucocytosis is a feature of many conditions including pregnancy, severe exercise and myocardial infarction. Megaloblastic anaemia and Felty's syndrome (rheumatoid arthritis, splenomegaly and lymphadenopathy) cause neutropenia.

11. (*a, b, d*)
Agranulocytosis is characterized by infections and mouth ulceration (hence dysphagia). Constitutional symptoms and delayed wound healing are common. Localized but not generalized lymphadenopathy is associated with specific infections (e.g. cervical lymphadenopathy with mouth ulcers).

12. (*b, c, e*)
Thrombocythaemia (increase in the numbers of circulating platelets) is not a recognized feature of either corticosteroid therapy or mycoplasma infections.

13. (*b, c, d, e*)
The fall in haemoglobin concentration after haemorrhage is dependent on haemodilution (reflected by a fall in PCV) and this does not usually occur for several hours. After such haemorrhage immature red cells often enter the circulation (polychromatic cells) and the platelet and neutrophil count increases.

14. (*a, c*)
Iron deficiency is associated with pallor, koilonychia and dysphagia (Plummer–Vinson syndrome). Grey discoloration of the skin is seen in haemochromatosis in which there is increased total body iron. Peripheral neuropathy is a feature of B_{12} deficiency.

15. Vitamin B_{12} deficiency occurs in

a. Pork tape-worm infestation (Taenia solium)
b. Crohn's disease
c. Bacterial contamination of the small bowel
d. Zollinger–Ellison syndrome
e. Gastrectomy

16. Pernicious anaemia is associated with the following:

a. Microcytic anaemia
b. Abnormal terminal ileum on barium meal
c. Hyperchlorhydria
d. Lemon-yellow skin discoloration
e. Petechial haemorrhages

17. Folic acid deficiency is

a. Rarely due to dietary deficiency.
b. Associated with treatment with phenytoin.
c. Complicated by subacute combined degeneration of the spinal cord in a minority of cases.
d. A recognized complication of pregnancy.
e. Associated with intrinsic factor antibodies.

18. The following are typical of haemolytic anaemia

a. Bilirubin present in the urine
b. Urobilinogen in the urine
c. Gallstones
d. Macrocytosis
e. Splenomegaly

19. In sickle-cell anaemia

a. Oesteoarthritis of the hips is a recognized feature.
b. Splenomegaly is more prominent with age.
c. Deformity of the skull is a recognized feature.
d. Severe abdominal pain is a recognized complaint.
e. The direct Coombs test is positive.

Answers overleaf

15. (*b, c, e*)
The commonest cause of vitamin B_{12} deficiency is pernicious anaemia. However, diminished vitamin B_{12} absorption due to gastrectomy (absence of intrinsic factor) or terminal ileum damage due to Crohn's disease also produce vitamin B_{12} deficiency. The fish tape-worm (Diphyllobothrium latum) and certain bacteria utilize vitamin B_{12} for their own metabolism.

16. (*d, e*)
Pernicious anaemia is due to B_{12} deficiency and is associated with achlorhydria and deficiency of gastric intrinsic factor (frequently with circulating intrinsic factor antibodies). It presents as a megaloblastic anaemia and there may be lemon-yellow discoloration of the skin (secondary to mild haemolysis), glossitis, neurological symptoms and petechial haemorrhages.

17. (*b, d*)
Folic acid deficiency is commonly due to a poor diet particularly at times of increased requirements (e.g. pregnancy). Certain drugs like phenytoin antagonize the action of folic acid. Subacute combined degeneration of the cord is a feature of vitamin B_{12} deficiency.

18. (*b, c, d, e*)
Haemolytic anaemia is associated with rapid red cell turnover and thus there is an increase in unconjugated bilirubin in the blood and urobilinogen in the urine. Obstructive jaundice very occasionally develops secondary to pigment gallstones. Macrocytosis and splenomegaly are typical findings.

19. (*a, c, d*)
Skeletal abnormalities with sickle-cell anaemia are common and include the skull and arthritis of the hips. Because of recurrent infarctions (one reason for abdominal pain) the spleen size shrinks with age and is frequently not palpable in affected adults. The Coombs test is positive in autoimmune haemolytic anaemias.

20. Which of the following statements about haemolytic anaemias are correct?

a. Thalassaemia is due to hereditary deficiency of glucose-6-phosphate dehydrogenase.
b. Methaemalbumin is a recognized feature of severe haemolysis.
c. Spherocytosis is associated with a positive Coombs test.
d. Erythroblastosis fetalis is due to neonatal septicaemia.
e. Increased osmotic fragility of red cells is characteristic of favism.

21. Which of the following statements about acute myeloblastic leukaemia are correct?

a. Is more common in children than adults.
b. Bony tenderness is a recognized symptom.
c. At least 70 per cent of patients survive 5 years.
d. Lymph node enlargement is a prominent feature.
e. Necrotic mouth ulceration is characteristic.

22. In acute lymphoblastic leukaemia

a. Remission can be induced in more than half of patients.
b. Central nervous system involvement occurs early in the course of the disease.
c. Subarachnoid haemorrhage is a recognized complication.
d. Fever is usually due to unusual infections.
e. Diagnosis can always be made on the routine peripheral blood film.

23. Recognized features of chronic myeloid leukaemia include

a. A male predominance
b. Moderate increase in white-cell count (up to $20\,000 \times 10^9$/l)
c. Massive splenomegaly
d. Decreased leucocyte alkaline phosphatase activity
e. Large numbers of myeloblasts in the peripheral blood

Answers overleaf

20. (*b*)

Thalassaemia is due to an hereditary haemoglobinopathy; glucose-6-phosphate deficiency is the cause of favism. Severe haemolysis is associated with plasma methaemalbumin, haemoglobinuria and haemosiderinuria. Increased osmotic fragility is a feature of spherocytosis while Coombs test is used to diagnose acquired autoimmune haemolytic anaemia. Erythroblastosis fetalis (haemolytic disease of the newborn) is most commonly due to rhesus incompatibility (passage of rhesus antibodies across the placenta).

21. (*b, e*)

Acute myeloblastic leukaemia is commoner in adults and its prognosis is worse than childhood lymphoblastic leukaemia. Necrotic mouth ulcers are a common presenting feature; later, exquisite bony tenderness may occur. Lymphadenopathy although occasionally present is not a prominent feature of this disease.

22. (*a, c*)

Acute lymphoblastic leukaemia is associated with haemorrhage (including subarachnoid); fever is also common and usually secondary to common pyogenic organisms. The diagnosis of an acute leukaemia can usually be made on the peripheral film, but marrow investigation and special staining techniques are required to be sure of the cell type. Central nervous system symptoms occur late in the disease.

23. (*c, d*)

Chronic myeloid leukaemia has an equal sex incidence and is characterized by very high white-cell counts (only occasional myeloblasts) and massive splenomegaly. The leucocyte alkaline phosphatase activity is very low.

24. Recognized features of chronic lymphatic leukaemia include

a. Equal sex incidence
b. Herpes zoster infections
c. Pruritus
d. Large numbers of immature lymphocytes on the peripheral blood film
e. Very poor prognosis

25. In myelofibrosis

a. Hepatomegaly without splenomegaly is a rare but well-recognized presentation.
b. Marrow aspiration usually yields a 'dry tap'.
c. Death usually occurs within 1 year of diagnosis.
d. The Philadelphia chromosome (Ph1) is present in 90 per cent of cases.
e. Pneumocystis pneumonia is a characteristic complication.

26. Hodgkin's disease

a. Has maximal incidence in early adult life.
b. Typically presents with painful lymphadenopathy.
c. Is characterized by multinucleate cells (Sternberg–Reed cells).
d. May be complicated by fever.
e. Bone marrow involvement is present in most cases.

27. Purpura may result from

a. Thrombocytopenia
b. Bacterial endocarditis
c. Vitamin D deficiency
d. Old age
e. Pernicious anaemia

Answers overleaf

24. (*b, c*)
In contrast to chronic myeloid, chronic lymphatic leukaemia is commonest in elderly men. There is impairment of both humoral and cellular immunity which predisposes patients to many infections including herpes zoster. The peripheral blood film consists mainly of mature lymphocytes. Pruritus is a recognized feature and the overall prognosis is between 1 and 10 years.

25. (*b*)
Myelofibrosis which has a prognosis measured in years is characterized by massive splenomegaly. Because of the marrow fibrosis aspiration often results in a 'dry tap' and thus a trephine biopsy is usually needed. The Philadelphia chromosome is a feature of chronic myeloid leukaemia. Pneumocystis pneumonia is not common although other infections are frequently encountered.

26. (*a, c, d*)
Hodgkin's disease has a maximal incidence in early adult life and is characterized by Sternberg–Reed cells. Painless lymphadenopathy is the commonest presentation and may be associated with constitutional symptoms (e.g. fever, lassitude and weight loss). Examination of the bone marrow is often normal.

27. (*a, b, d, e*)
Purpura is due to increased capillary permeability from various causes including thrombocytopenia, old age, pernicious anaemia, bacterial endocarditis and vitamin C (not D) deficiency.

28. Which of the following statements about purpura are correct?

a. Cutaneous purpura may be induced by corticosteroid therapy.
b. Purpuric spots blanch on firm pressure.
c. Moderate splenomegaly is a typical feature of idiopathic thrombocytopenic purpura.
d. Purpuric spots on the head are a feature of severe coughing bouts in young children.
e. The Henoch–Schönlein syndrome is related to haemolytic streptococcal infections.

29. Scurvy

a. Is due to vitamin E deficiency.
b. Is typically associated with bleeding spongy gums.
c. Petechiae characteristically cluster around hair follicles.
d. The legs are usually unaffected.
e. Haemarthrosis is common.

30. Which of the following statements relating to haemophilia are correct?

a. It is due to factor VII deficiency.
b. Male haemophiliacs transmit the carrier state to all their daughters.
c. Bleeding time is prolonged.
d. Bleeding into large joints is characteristic.
e. The carrier state is associated with a very mild bleeding tendency.

Answers overleaf

28. (*a, d, e*)
Many drugs can induce a purpuric rash either by increasing capillary fragility (e.g. corticosteroids) or by thrombocytopenia due to marrow damage. Purpuric spots never blanch on pressure. Purpuric spots on the head occasionally occur after very severe coughing bouts in early childhood. Splenomegaly is an unusual feature of idiopathic thrombocytopenic purpura.

29. (*b, c*)
Scurvy is due to vitamin C (not E) deficiency and is characterized by extensive ecchymoses particularly on the legs. Petechiae tend to be around hair follicles and spongy gums are only seen if the patient has teeth. Haemorrhage into muscle occurs but haemarthroses are uncommon.

30. (*b, d*)
Haemophilia (due to factor VIII deficiency) is a sex-linked hereditary disease and all the daughters of an affected man are asymptomatic carriers. The bleeding time is normal (this depends on capillary contractility) and clotting time is prolonged. Haemarthroses are very common and may lead to severe deformity.

1. A woman aged 62 years gave a 3-month history of dyspnoea, palpitations, tiredness, indigestion, tingling in the feet and unsteadiness of gait. Examination revealed pallor, impaired vibration and joint position sense in the legs, absent ankle reflexes and extensor plantar responses.

a. What is the most likely diagnosis?
b. Give the results of two investigations which would help confirm this diagnosis.

2. A 32-year-old man complained of lassitude and weight loss. Examination revealed pallor, painless cervical lymphadenopathy and splenomegaly. The chest radiograph revealed paratracheal lymph nodes.

a. What is the probable diagnosis?
b. Name three other possible clinical features.
c. How would you confirm the diagnosis?

3. A 60-year-old man complained of fatigue, weakness, weight loss and attacks of sweating. He was pale; there were superficial bruises and he had massive splenomegaly.

a. Give the most likely diagnosis.
b. Give two typical abnormalities in the blood.
c. What is the associated chromosomal abnormality?

4. A 55-year-old woman developed chronic backache, anaemia and recurrent chest infections. She then noticed a painful swelling on her left clavicle which enlarged over a period of a few weeks. Her haemoglobin was 8 g/dl and erythrocyte sedimentation rate was 115 mm in the first hour.

a. What is the probable diagnosis and how would you confirm it?
b. What is the cause of the swelling on the clavicle?
c. List two complications of this condition.

Answers overleaf

1. *a*. Pernicious anaemia
b. (i) Megaloblastic marrow
(ii) Low serum B_{12} level

2. *a*. Lymphoma (e.g. Hodgkin's disease)
b. (i) Pyrexia
(ii) Pruritus
(iii) Jaundice
c. Histology of affected tissue

3. *a*. Chronic myeloid leukaemia
b. (i) Normocytic normochromic anaemia
(ii) White-cell count of more than $100\,000 \times 10^9$/l
c. Philadelphia chromosome

4. *a*. (i) Multiple myeloma
(ii) Plasma protein electrophoresis
b. Plasmacytoma
c. (i) Renal failure
(ii) Pathological fractures

Arrange the following associations into their correct pairs:

1. *A*. Oesophageal webs
   B. Generalized lymphadenopathy
   C. Stony hard lymphadenopathy
   D. Painful lymphadenopathy
   E. Haemarthroses

   a. Carcinoma of the bronchus
   b. Pyogenic infections
   c. Glandular fever
   d. Haemophilia
   e. Severe iron deficiency anaemia

2. *A*. Massive splenomegaly
   B. Minor splenomegaly
   C. Optic atrophy
   D. Retinal vein engorgement
   E. Fundal haemorrhages

   a. Polycythaemia vera
   b. Myelofibrosis
   c. Sudden gastric haemorrhage
   d. Glandular fever
   e. Vitamin B_{12} deficiency

3. *A*. Koilonychia
   B. Gum hypertrophy
   C. Spongy and bleeding gums
   D. Angular stomatitis
   E. Tonsilar enlargement

   a. Vitamin C deficiency
   b. Ariboflavinosis
   c. Lymphosarcoma
   d. Acute leukaemia
   e. Severe iron deficiency

4. *A*. Raised PCV
   B. Megaloblasts in the blood
   C. Basophilic stippling
   D. Rouleaux formation
   E. Howell–Jolly bodies

   a. Multiple myeloma
   b. Post-splenectomy
   c. Polycythaemia vera
   d. Folate deficiency
   e. Lead poisoning

5. *A*. Leucocytosis
   B. Eosinophilia
   C. Thrombocythaemia
   D. Lymphopenia
   E. Total leucopenia

   a. Polycythemia vera
   b. Felty's syndrome
   c. Myocardial infarction
   d. Viral infections
   e. Asthma

6. *A*. Macrocytic anaemia
   B. Microcytic anaemia
   C. Skull deformity
   D. Red-cell osmotic fragility
   E. Positive Coombs test

   a. Iron deficiency
   b. Folate deficiency
   c. Autoimmune haemolytic anaemia
   d. Sickle-cell anaemia
   e. Spherocytosis

Answers overleaf

1. *A......e*
B......c
C......a
D......b
E......d

2. *A......b*
B......d
C......e
D......a
E......c

3. *A......e*
B......d
C......a
D......b
E......c

4. *A......c*
B......d
C......e
D......a
E......b

5. *A......c*
B......e
C......a
D......d
E......b

6. *A......b*
B......a
C......d
D......e
E......c

7. *A*. Philadelphia chromosome
B. Hypercalcaemia
C. Sternberg–Reed cells
D. Factor VIII deficiency
E. Post-streptococcal infection

a. Haemophilia
b. Henoch–Schönlein syndrome
c. Chronic myeloid leukaemia
d. Myeloma
e. Hodgkin's disease

Answers overleaf

7. *A*......*c*
B......*d*
C......*e*
D......*a*
E......*b*

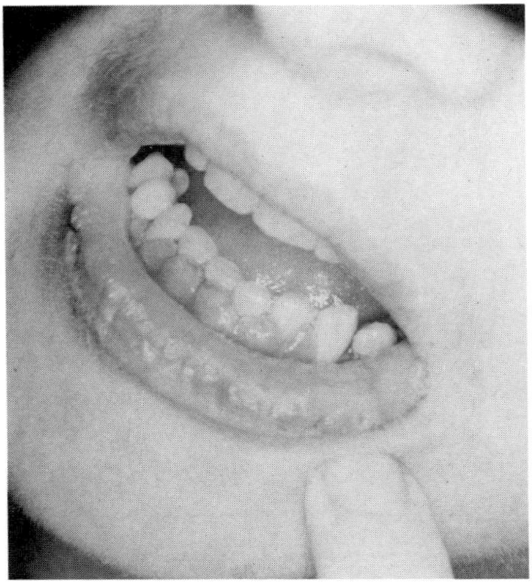

Fig. 8.1
a. What abnormality is shown?
b. Give two possible causes.

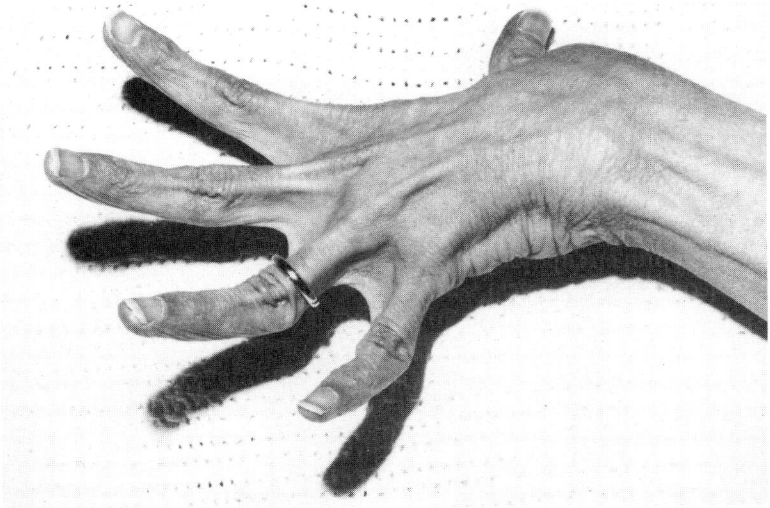

Fig. 8.2
a. What abnormality is displayed here?
b. With which rare syndrome may it be associated?

Answers overleaf

Fig. 8.1
a. Gum hypertrophy
b. Phenytoin therapy; leukaemia

Fig. 8.2
a. Hyperextensibility of joints
b. Ehlers–Danlos syndrome

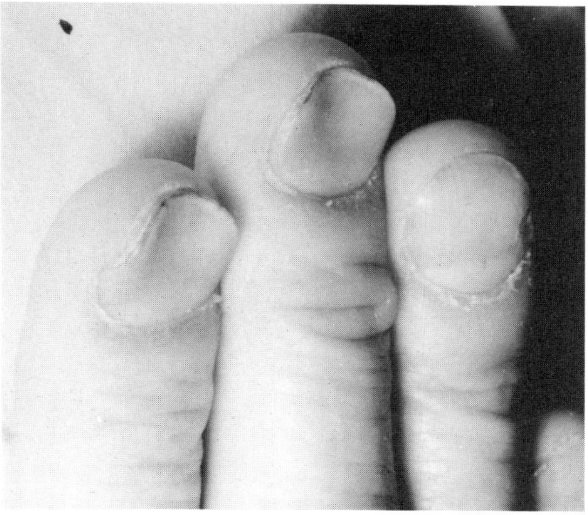

Fig. 8.3
a. What name is given to this appearance?
b. With what condition is it associated?

Answers overleaf

Fig. 8.3
a. Koilonychia
b. Iron deficiency

The Skeletal System

(Refer to Chapter 9 in *Symptoms and Signs in Clinical Medicine*, 11th edition, p. 318.)

1. An increased temperature over the affected part is a feature of

a. Paget's disease
b. Charcot's joint
c. Rheumatoid arthritis
d. Osteoarthrosis
e. Gout

2. Small peripheral joints are involved predominantly and early in

a. Rheumatic fever
b. Gout
c. Rheumatoid arthritis
d. Infective arthritis
e. Ankylosing spondylitis

3. The range of movement is 80° or more for the following:

a. Shoulder flexion
b. Shoulder adduction
c. Ulnar deviation of the wrist
d. Hip external rotation
e. Toe flexion (interphalangeal joint)

4. The alkaline phosphatase is commonly raised in

a. Paget's disease
b. Osteomalacia
c. Bone metastases, from breast carcinoma
d. Osteoporosis
e. Rheumatoid arthritis

5. Paget's disease

a. Mainly affects the elderly.
b. May be complicated by cardiac failure.
c. Can produce paraplegia.
d. Produces a 'sabre' tibia.
e. Is accompanied by bone pains.

Answers overleaf

1. (*a, c, e*)
Charcot's joint and oesteoarthrosis are degenerative arthropathies, whereas rheumatoid arthritis and gout are inflammatory and therefore accompanied by a raised temperature over the affected joint. Increased blood flow through actively proliferating bone accounts in Paget's disease for the increased temperature of the overlying tissues.

2. (*b, c*)
Gout characteristically first affects the great toe joints and rheumatoid arthritis the small joints of the hands and feet. Rheumatic fever and infective arthritis favour the large joints and ankylosing spondylitis the proximal joints (spine, sacroiliac and hip).

3. (*a, e*)
Shoulder flexion attains 180° and toe flexion 90°. The others are less than 80° (shoulder adduction 45°, ulnar deviation 30° and hip external rotation 60°).

4. (*a, b, c*)
Alkaline phosphatase is a bone enzyme which is excreted in the bile. Blood levels may be raised in certain diffuse bone disorders (but not in cases of simple osteoporosis) and liver diseases.

5. (*a, b, c, e*)
Increased blood flow through actively proliferating bone may lead to high output cardiac failure and bone pains. Overgrowth of bone can result in compression of the spinal cord, enlargement of the head, and broadening and bowing of long bones such as the tibia. The bowed anterior border of the tibia is sharp rather than broadened in the rare 'sabre' tibia of syphilis.

6. Permanent sequelae of rheumatic fever include

a. Joint deformities
b. Aortic valve disease
c. Huntington's chorea
d. Mitral stenosis
e. Constrictive pericarditis

7. There is a recognized association between rheumatoid arthritis and

a. Heberden's nodes
b. Urethritis
c. Anaemia
d. Lung nodules
e. Ulnar deviation of the fingers

8. Ankylosing spondylitis

a. Mainly affects older women.
b. Commonly involves the sacroiliac joint.
c. Is usually painless.
d. May limit chest expansion.
e. May be accompanied by aortic stenosis.

9. The following diagnostic tests are appropriate:

a. Antistreptolysin titre: for rheumatoid arthritis
b. Human lymphocyte antigen B_{27}: for ankylosing spondylitis
c. Serum uric acid: for Reiter's syndrome
d. Alkaline phosphatase: for gout
e. Wassermann reaction: for Charcot's joints

10. A neuropathic joint may result from

a. Tabes dorsalis
b. Motor neurone disease
c. Syringomyelia
d. Diabetes
e. Hemiplegia

Answers overleaf

6. (*b, d*)
Mitral and aortic valve disease are important permanent sequelae of rheumatic fever. Arthritis, pericarditis and Sydenham's chorea are all transient disorders occurring during the acute phase of the illness. (Huntington's chorea is a rare inherited disease unrelated to rheumatism.)

7. (*c, d, e*)
Heberden's nodes (bony nodules over the distal interphalangeal joints) are a feature of osteoarthritis. The nodules of rheumatoid disease are not bony and may occur in the lung as well as in subcutaneous tissues. Urethritis occurs in Reiter's syndrome, not in rheumatoid disease.

8. (*b, d*)
Ankylosing spondylitis most often presents in young men with low back pain due to inflammation of the sacroiliac joints. Ankylosis of costovertebral as well as intervertebral joints leads to impaired chest expansion. It is occasionally associated with aortic regurgitation.

9. (*b, e*)
The antistreptolysin titre is used for the detection of recent streptococcal infection in the diagnosis of rheumatic fever. The serum uric acid is raised in cases of gout, while serum alkaline phosphatase is raised in certain diffuse disorders of bone. The Wassermann reaction would be an appropriate test in Reiter's syndrome (as well as in Charcot's joints) since this is venereal, though not syphilitic, in origin.

10. (*a, c, d*)
A neuropathic joint results from loss of the protection provided for the joint by deep pain sensation as in tabes, syringomyelia and diabetic neuropathy. It cannot result from purely motor conditions such as motor neurone disease and hemiplegia.

11. These observations may help to distinguish osteoarthritis from rheumatoid arthritis

a. The ESR
b. The presence of arthritic changes in the finger joints
c. The temperature of the affected joint
d. The finding of subcutaneous nodules
e. The age of presentation

12. Gout

a. May be inherited.
b. Can be precipitated by thiazide diuretics.
c. Occurs in acute attacks.
d. May lead to renal failure.
e. Affects men more than women.

Answers overleaf

11. (*a, c, d, e*)
Rheumatoid disease, unlike osteoarthritis, is an inflammatory disorder so that, at least in the acute stage of the disease, the affected joints are hot and the ESR is raised. Both conditions can involve the finger joints, but subcutaneous nodules are found only in rheumatoid disease. Rheumatoid arthritis usually presents in early adult life, oesteoarthritis in older patients.

12. (All correct)
These statements are all true for gout.

1. A 42-year-old man was found at a routine medical examination to have albuminuria and a blood pressure of 160/90. Apart from an episode of cellulitis in the foot, his previous health had been good. His father died from a stroke at the age of 54 and his brother suffered from arthritis; the remainder of his family was well. The blood pressure fell to 130/70 when treatment with bendrofluazide was started. However, he then suddenly developed a painful swelling of the left knee which settled after a few days' rest but recurred a few weeks later when he sought medical advice.

a. What is the most likely diagnosis?
b. List three diagnostic signs which might be present.
c. What investigation might confirm the diagnosis?

2. A young man complained of some stiffness of his lower back. On examination there was tenderness over the sacroiliac joints but no other abnormality.

a. What diagnosis should be considered?
b. Name two complications of this disorder.
c. Name two relevant diagnostic investigations.

Answers overleaf

1. *a*. Gout
b. (i) Signs of joint inflammation (especially big toe)
(ii) Tophi in ear
(iii) Urates extruded around joints
c. Raised serum urate

2. *a*. Ankylosing spondylitis
b. (i) Iritis
(ii) Aortic incompetence
c. (i) X-ray of lumbar spine and pelvis
(ii) HLA status

Arrange the following associations into their correct pairs:

1. *A*. Terminal interphalangeal joints
B. Sacroiliac joints
C. Proximal interphalangeal joints
D. Weight-bearing joints
E. First metatarso-phalangeal joint

a. Psoriatic arthritis
b. Rheumatoid arthritis
c. Gout
d. Ankylosing spondylitis
e. Osteoarthritis

2. *A*. Vitamin D deficiency
B. Impaired urate metabolism
C. Diabetic neuropathy
D. β-Haemolytic streptococci
E. Multiple myeloma

a. Charcot's joint
b. Hypercalcaemia
c. Rheumatic fever
d. Gout
e. Osteomalacia

3. *A*. Bow legs
B. Erythema marginatum
C. Lung nodules
D. Reduced chest expansion
E. Non-bacterial urethritis

a. Rheumatic fever
b. Paget's disease
c. Rheumatoid disease
d. Reiter's syndrome
e. Ankylosing spondylitis

4. *A*. Post-menopausal kyphosis
B. Proximal muscle stiffness
C. Hypertension
D. Heberden's nodes
E. Aortic regurgitation

a. Osteoarthritis
b. Gout
c. Ankylosing spondylitis
d. Osteoporosis
e. Polymyalgia rheumatica

5. *A*. Raised antistreptolysin titre
B. (HLA) B_{27}
C. Raised serum uric acid
D. Positive antinuclear factor
E. High alkaline phosphatase

a. Gout
b. Systemic lupus erythematosus
c. Rheumatic fever
d. Ankylosing spondylitis
e. Paget's disease

Answers overleaf

1. *A*......*a*
B......*d*
C......*b*
D......*e*
E......*c*

2. *A*......*e*
B......*d*
C......*a*
D......*c*
E......*b*

3. *A*......*b*
B......*a*
C......*c*
D......*e*
E......*d*

4. *A*......*d*
B......*e*
C......*b*
D......*a*
E......*c*

5. *A*......*c*
B......*d*
C......*a*
D......*b*
E......*e*

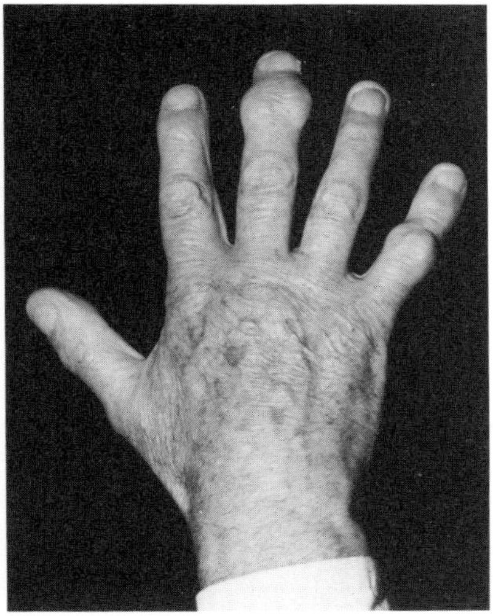

Fig. 9.1
a. What is the diagnosis?
b. Give two signs to be found outside the joints.

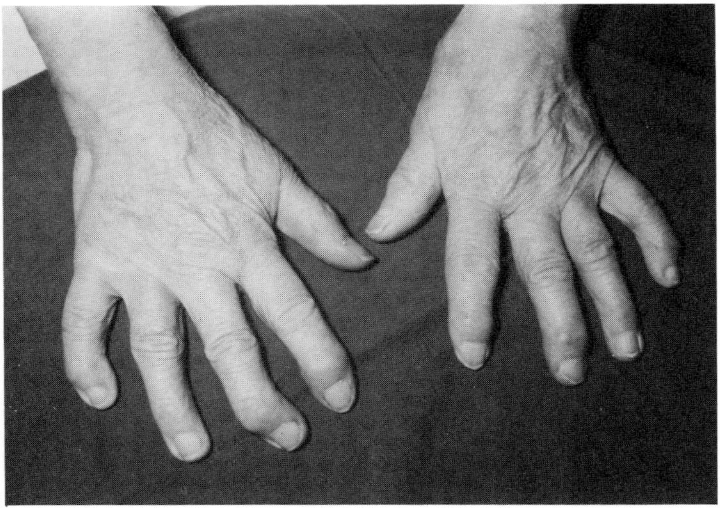

Fig. 9.2
a. What abnormality is shown?
b. What may it signify?

Answers overleaf

Fig. 9.1
a. Gout
b. Cutaneous tophi (ears especially); hypertension

Fig. 9.2
a. Heberden's nodes
b. Osteoarthritis

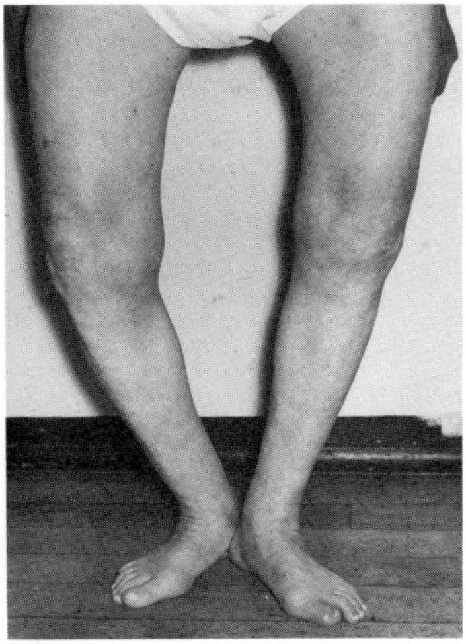

Fig. 9.3
a. Who first described this condition?
b. Why might this patient have complained of deafness?

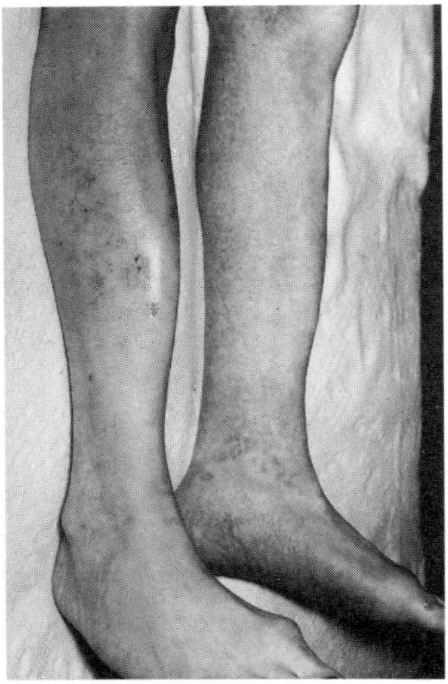

Fig. 9.4
a. To which offensive weapon is this appearance likened?
b. What is the cause?

Answers overleaf

Fig. 9.3
a. Sir James Paget (surgeon to St Bartholemew's Hospital, London)
b. Because bony overgrowth may compress the 8th nerve in the auditory canal

Fig. 9.4
a. Sabre (tibia)
b. Syphilis

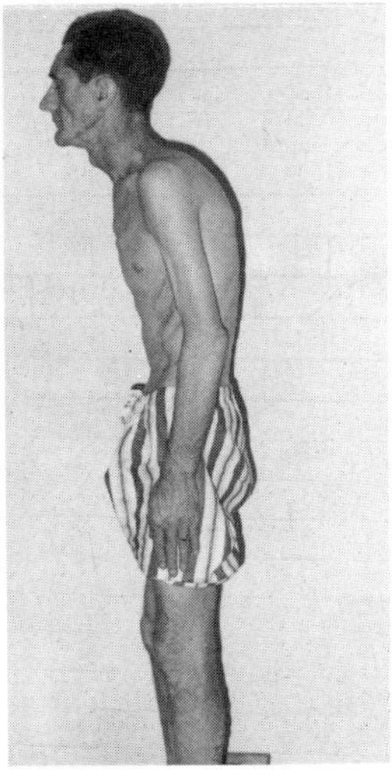

Fig. 9.5
a. This shows the characteristic posture of which joint disorder?
b. Which are the three most commonly affected groups of joints?

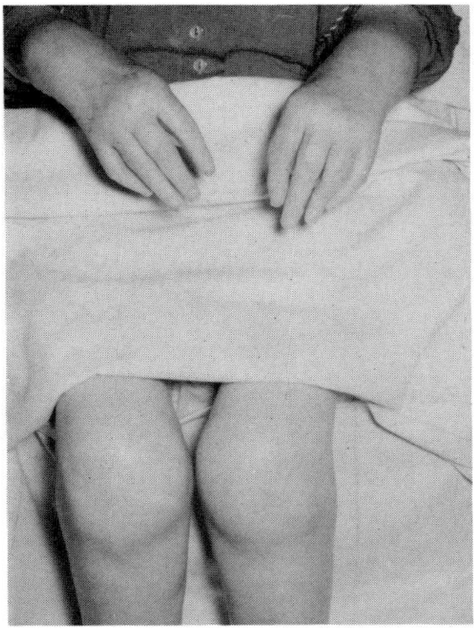

Fig. 9.6
a. What is the diagnosis?
b. List three lesions which might be found outside the joints.

Answers overleaf

Fig. 9.5
a. Ankylosing spondylitis
b. Sacroiliac; intervertebral, costovertebral

Fig. 9.6
a. Rheumatoid arthritis
b. Ocular lesions (iritis, scleritis); pulmonary lesions (nodules, fibrosis, pleurisy); subcutaneous nodules

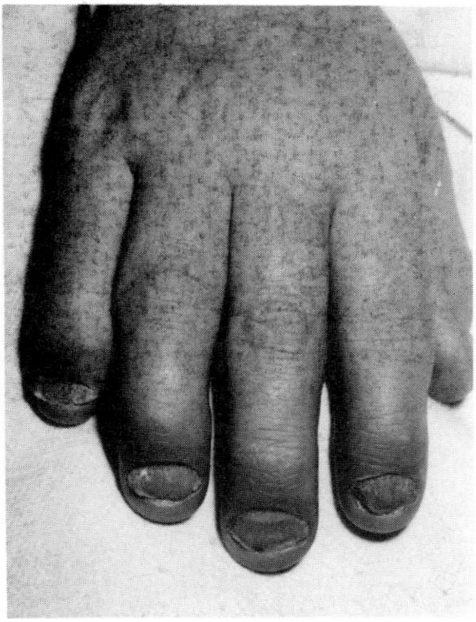

Fig. 9.7
a. What abnormalities are shown?
b. What might inspection of the remainder of the body reveal?

Answers overleaf

Fig. 9.7
a. Scarred, pitted nails and swelling of terminal interphalangeal joints
b. The skin lesions of psoriasis

The Nervous System

(Refer to Chapter 10 in *Symptoms and Signs in Clinical Medicine*, 11th edition, p. 338.)

1. There is a recognized association between facial paralysis and

a. Loss of taste on the posterior third of the tongue
b. Hyperacusis
c. Herpetic eruption on the pinna of the ear
d. Ptosis
e. Corneal ulceration

2. Right homonymous hemianopia is caused by lesions of

a. The retina
b. The right optic nerve
c. The optic chiasma
d. The left optic tract
e. The left optic radiations

3. In complete paralysis of the 3rd nerve

a. The pupil is dilated.
b. The pupil on the affected side shows a normal consensual response to light.
c. The pupil does not react to accommodation.
d. There is ptosis.
e. There is internal strabismus.

4. Nystagmus commonly accompanies

a. Congenital blindness
b. Vertigo
c. Vestibular lesions
d. Third nerve paralysis
e. Cerebellar disorders

5. The trigeminal nerve mediates

a. The corneal reflex
b. The gag reflex
c. The jaw jerk
d. The pupil response to accommodation
e. The ciliospinal reflex

Answers overleaf

1. (*b, c, e*)
The 7th nerve carries the chorda tympani which conveys the sense of taste from the anterior two-thirds of the tongue. The 7th nerve supplies the stapedius muscle which damps the vibration of the eardrum so that noises are louder if the muscle is paralysed. Herpes zoster affecting the geniculate ganglion causes facial paralysis and herpetic lesions on the ear. Facial paralysis prevents the eye from closing (not opening) and thus predisposes to corneal ulceration.

2. (*d, e*)
A right homonymous hemianopia is loss of vision in the right half of the visual field due to interruption of fibres from the temporal half of the left retina and nasal half of the right retina. These two groups of fibres run together only in the left optic tract, radiation and occipital cortex and cannot be involved together in or anterior to the chiasma.

3. (*a, c, d*)
In complete 3rd nerve paralysis, the pupil is dilated and fixed showing no direct or consensual reaction to light and no reaction to accommodation. There is ptosis and paralysis of all ocular movements except outwards (6th nerve) and slight rotation (intortion) when attempting to look downwards and medially (4th nerve); there is therefore an external strabismus.

4. (*a, b, c, e*)
Nystagmus may result from visual, vestibular or cerebellar disorders and it invariably accompanies true vertigo, but it is not caused by lesions of the oculomotor nerves.

5. (*a, c*)
The trigeminal nerve provides the afferent arc for the corneal reflex and the afferent and efferent arcs for the jaw jerk. The gag reflex is mediated by the 9th or 10th nerve. Constriction of the pupil on accommodation is mediated by the 3rd nerve, while dilatation of the pupils in response to pinching the neck (ciliospinal reflex) is due to stimulation of the cervical sympathetic.

6. Abnormal dilatation of one pupil may be due to

a. Mydriatic drugs
b. A myotonic pupil (Adie–Holmes syndrome)
c. Paralysis of cervical sympathetic
d. Subdural haematoma
e. Diabetes

7. Trigeminal neuralgia

a. Is commoner in older patients.
b. Affects men more than women.
c. Is a dull, aching pain.
d. Tends to be sudden and transient.
e. May be complicated by sensory loss in the face.

8. Which of the following statements are true for unilateral conductive deafness?

a. The cause may lie in the middle ear.
b. It may complicate Menière's syndrome.
c. It occurs with lesions of the 8th nerve.
d. The sound of a tuning fork applied to the forehead is heard best in the normal ear (Weber's test).
e. Bone conduction from a tuning fork is heard better than air conduction (Rinne's test).

9. Lesions of the upper motor neurone may result in

a. Inability to close the eye
b. Conjugate deviation of the eyes
c. Brisk jaw jerk
d. Dysarthria
e. Fasciculation of the tongue

10. The following are characteristic of disturbance of the higher cerebral centres:

a. Dyslexia
b. Dysarthria
c. Dysphonia
d. Dysgraphia
e. Dysphasia

Answers overleaf

6. (*a, b, d*)
A mydriatic drug is one which dilates the pupil and may be used to facilitate ophthalmoscopy. The myotonic pupil is of normal diameter or dilated, reacts sluggishly to accommodation but not to light. Cervical sympathetic paralysis and diabetes cause pupil restriction. Dilatation of one or both pupils is a grave sign in patients with subdural haematoma or other space-occupying intracranial lesions.

7. (*a, d*)
Trigeminal neuralgia usually affects older women. It is sharp, sudden and transient. It may be triggered by touching the skin of the face, but there is no sensory loss.

8. (*a, e*)
The term 'condutive deafness' implies impaired conduction between the external meatus and the receptor organs of the inner ear. It may, therefore, result from obstruction to the external meatus or disease of the drum or middle ear, but not from disorders of the inner ear itself (as in Menière's syndrome) nor of the 8th nerve. Bone-conducted sound is heard better than air-conducted sound and may actually be louder in the affected ear (due to exclusion of background noise).

9. (*b, c, d*)
Lesions of the upper motor neurone supplying the 7th nerve nucleus cause paresis of the lower part of the face only. Upper motor neurone lesions impair conjugate movements, not individual muscles. Bilateral upper motor neurone lesions affecting bulbar (medullary) nuclei cause a brisk jaw jerk, dysphagia and dysarthria. The tongue may be small and spastic but wasting and fasciculation occur only with lower motor neurone lesions.

10. (*a, d, e*)
Dyslexia, dysgraphia and dysphasia refer respectively to difficulties in reading, writing and speech of central origin. Dysarthria is difficulty in execution of speech by the oral musculature, while dysphonia is difficulty in producing a laryngeal sound.

11. The causes of papilloedema include

a. Hypertension
b. Hypercapnia
c. Glaucoma
d. Multiple sclerosis
e. Cerebral tumour

12. Hypertensive retinopathy is characterized by

a. Optic atrophy
b. Microaneurysms
c. Proliferative retinopathy
d. Haemorrhages and exudates
e. Venous nipping at arterial crossings

13. Which of the following statements are true of non-paralytic (concomitant) strabismus?

a. Is commonly present from childhood.
b. Is accompanied by diplopia.
c. Vision of the affected eye is impaired.
d. Visual axis is unchanged on ocular movement.
e. Range of ocular movements is restricted.

14. Ataxia may result from disorders of the

a. Cerebellum
b. Basal ganglia
c. Spinothalamic tract
d. Dorsal columns
e. Internal capsule

15. Lesions of the internal capsule may produce

a. Contralateral hemiplegia
b. Parkinsonism
c. Contralateral hemianaesthesia
d. Ipsilateral homonymous hemianopia
e. Aphasia

Answers overleaf

11. (*a, b, e*)
Papilloedema results from malignant (accelerated) hypertension, from the intense vasodilatory effects of carbon dioxide excess (hypercapnia) and from cerebral tumour or other space-occupying lesions. Glaucoma causes optic atrophy from raised intraocular tension, while multiple sclerosis also causes optic atrophy but may present with an optic neuritis, in which there is redness and blurring of the disc but no true papilloedema.

12. (*d, e*)
Although optic atrophy may rarely follow long-standing papilloedema in malignant hypertension, this is not a characteristic finding. Microaneurysms and proliferative retinopathy are typical features of diabetic retinopathy.

13. (*a, c, d*)
Adaptation to concomitant strabismus from early childhood causes inhibition of visual impulses from the affected eye and thus no diplopia. There is an imbalance of opposing muscles rather than paralysis so that the visual axis remains constant and the range of movements unrestricted.

14. (*a, d, e*)
Ataxia may be due to motor incoordination of cerebellar origin or to lack of sensory information conveyed by the dorsal columns and their central extensions through the internal capsule.

15. (*a, c, e*)
The internal capsule conveys the main motor, sensory and visual pathways between the cortex and the opposite side of the body. Complete interruption of these pathways therefore causes contralateral hemiplegia, hemianaesthesia and hemianopia. Aphasia also occurs if the lesion is on the left side.

16. The following are features of motor neurone disease:

a. Onset in later life
b. Muscle fasciculation
c. Extensor plantar responses
d. Wasting of the small muscles of the hands
e. Dysarthria

17. Lower motor neurone lesions are characterized by

a. Hypotonia
b. Clonus
c. Absent abdominal reflexes
d. Absent tendon reflexes
e. Muscle wasting

18. Choreiform movement

a. Is rhythmic.
b. Consists of repetition of the same movements.
c. May be predominantly unilateral.
d. Can be of rheumatic origin.
e. May be accompanied by cardiac murmurs.

19. Which of the following statements are true of peripheral neuropathy?

a. Paraesthesiae may precede physical signs.
b. The tendon reflexes are exaggerated.
c. It may result from thiamine deficiency.
d. There may be both sensory and motor deficits.
e. Diabetes is a very rare cause.

20. Parkinsonism is characterized by

a. High steppage gait
b. Intention tremor
c. Cog-wheel rigidity
d. Bradykinesia
e. Increased salivation

Answers overleaf

16. (All correct)
Motor neurone disease affects both the upper and lower motor neurones of the spinal cord and medulla.

17. (*a, d, e*)
Patella and ankle clonus are present only when the tendon reflexes are abnormally brisk due to an upper motor neurone lesion. The abdominal reflexes are mediated by the upper motor neurone and are absent if the pyramidal tract (or sensory arc of the reflex) is interrupted.

18. (*c, d, e*)
A rhythmic 'tremor' is characteristic of Parkinsonism, while repetitive movements are more suggestive of habit spasm or tics than of chorea. Rheumatic heart disease is sometimes associated with chorea.

19. (*a, c, d*)
Paraesthesiae are usually the earliest manifestation of a peripheral neuropathy. The signs may include both sensory and lower motor neurone loss with absent reflexes. Among the commonest causes in the world as a whole is thiamine deficiency and, in western countries, diabetes.

20. (*c, d, e*)
In Parkinsonism there is a shuffling ('festinating') gait; high stepping occurs when there is foot drop due to peripheral neuropathy. Unlike the intention tremor of cerebellar origin, Parkinsonian tremor tends to diminish on action.

21. Abolition of tendon reflexes is expected in

a. Brainstem lesions
b. Peripheral neuropathy
c. Lesions of the pyramidal tract
d. Diseases of the basal ganglia
e. Anterior horn cell lesions

22. In cases of hemiplegia

a. The cause is usually vascular.
b. The commonly affected artery is the anterior cerebral.
c. The upper face is predominantly affected.
d. The arm is usually weaker than the leg.
e. The abdominal reflexes are brisker on the paralysed side.

23. Radial nerve lesions may cause

a. Impaired adduction of the thumb
b. Paresis of digital extension
c. Loss of sensation over the dorsum of the thumb, index and middle fingers
d. Diminished biceps reflex
e. Wrist drop

24. Dystrophia myotonica

a. Is inherited as a sex-linked recessive characteristic.
b. Causes impaired muscle relaxation.
c. May be accompanied by testicular atrophy.
d. Predominantly affects the limb muscles.
e. Causes ptosis.

25. Myasthenia gravis

a. Is due to deficiency of anticholinesterase.
b. May be associated with hyperthyroidism.
c. Causes wasting of the shoulder girdle muscles.
d. Is worse at the beginning of the day.
e. Can be improved by cholinergic drugs.

Answers overleaf

21. (*b, e*)
Except in deep coma or spinal shock, the tendon reflexes are abolished only by lesions within the reflex arc, i.e. in the anterior or posterior horn cells, the peripheral nerves and their roots or in the muscles if these are grossly wasted.

22. (*a, d*)
The commonest cause of hemiplegia is a vascular lesion involving the middle cerebral artery supply to the internal capsule, where the arm fibres tend to be damaged more than those to the leg. Occlusion of the anterior cerebral artery causes paralysis of the leg alone, and cortical vascular lesions in general would have to be very extensive to affect the whole of one side (hemiplegia). The upper face and forehead are usually spared because of their bilateral pyramidal tract supply. The abdominal reflexes are abolished by disorders of the upper motor neurone.

23. (*b, e*)
The radial nerve supplies the triceps and extensors of the wrist and digits, but adduction of the thumb is mediated by the ulnar nerve. The radial nerve conveys sensation from the dorsum of the thumb, the median nerve from the dorsum of the index and middle fingers.

24. (*b, c, e*)
Dystrophia myotonica is transmitted by dominant inheritance. It is characterized by failure of muscle relaxation and wasting, especially of the facial musculature, with ptosis a striking feature. Baldness, cataract and testicular atrophy may also occur.

25. (*b, e*)
Myasthenia gravis is characterized by impairment of the mechanism whereby acetylcholine effects neuromuscular transmission. It is, therefore, not due to deficiency of anticholinesterase, but it can be improved by cholinergic drugs. Neuromuscular transmission is readily exhausted so that muscles tire as the day goes on. The condition is thought to be an autoimmune disorder in which the thyroid and thymus glands may also be involved.

26. Gross muscle wasting is a characteristic feature of

a. Myasthenia gravis
b. Upper motor neurone lesions
c. Parkinsonism
d. Cerebellar disorders
e. Motor neurone disease

27. Cerebellar disorders cause

a. Clonus
b. Nystagmus
c. Hypotonia
d. Sensory ataxia
e. Dysphasia

28. The spinothalamic tracts

a. Run in the anterolateral part of the spinal cord.
b. Decussate in the medulla.
c. Convey temperature sensation.
d. Reach the thalamus in the medial lemniscus.
e. Receive fibres from the anterior nerve root.

29. A parietal lobe tumour is likely to cause

a. Apraxia
b. Ataxia
c. Agnosia
d. Astereognosis
e. Aphasia

30. Paraesthesiae may be associated with

a. Peripheral neuropathy
b. Epilepsy
c. Hypoventilation
d. Cerebellar lesions
e. Local ischaemia

Answers overleaf

26. (*e*)
Wasting of muscles is usually gross only when the lower motor neurone is damaged or in cases of primary muscle disorders (the myopathies). It may also occur as a result of disuse (e.g. in the muscles moving a severely arthritic joint).

27. (*b, c*)
The cerebellum is responsible for the coordination of movements. Cerebellar disorders therefore result in intention tremor, motor ataxia and dysarthria ('staccato' speech). Upper motor neurone lesions cause clonus and dorsal column lesions sensory ataxia. Dysphasia refers to a speech defect of cerebral origin.

28. (*a, c, d*)
Nerve fibres conveying pain and temperature enter the spinal cord through the posterior nerve root, immediately cross over to enter the opposite spinothalamic tract and then travel, without further decussation, to the thalamus via the medial lemniscus. The anterior nerve root carries only motor fibres.

29. (*a, c, d, e*)
Ataxia is usually due to a cerebellar (motor) or dorsal column (sensory) lesion. Inability to perform complex movements (apraxia), sensory suppression (agnosia) and failure to identify objects by touch (astereognosis) are characteristic of parietal lesions, and speech defect (aphasia) may also occur.

30. (*a, b, e*)
Paraesthesiae (tingling sensations, pins and needles, numbness, etc.) may occur in all forms of peripheral neuropathy, as an aura in epilepsy and when arterial circulation to the part is impaired. They may also accompany the alkalotic tetany of hyperventilation.

31. Lesions of the nerve roots

a. Cause pain made worse by coughing.
b. May be due to herpes zoster.
c. Can result in loss of tendon reflexes.
d. Are a feature of poliomyelitis.
e. Cause ataxia.

32. The following signs are characteristic of cerebral cortical lesions:

a. Astereognosis
b. Loss of tactile discrimination
c. Dissociated anaesthesia
d. Loss of temperature discrimination
e. Grasp reflex

33. The following statements are true or false?

a. Thalamic lesions cause spontaneous pain.
b. Ipsilateral hemianaesthesia results from internal capsule stroke.
c. Root lesions cause segmental anaesthesia.
d. Central cord lesions produce dissociated anaesthesia.
e. Loss of proprioception indicates dorsal column disease.

34. Syringomyelia

a. Is due to obstruction to the flow of CSF.
b. Commonly causes muscle wasting in the legs.
c. May lead to Charcot joint changes in the arms.
d. Is characterized by dissociated anaesthesia.
e. May cause suspended anaesthesia.

35. Tabes dorsalis

a. Is due to a protozoal infection.
b. Causes ataxia.
c. Interferes with vesical reflexes.
d. Results in exaggerated tendon reflexes.
e. Causes patchy analgesia.

Answers overleaf

31. (*a, b, c*)
Lesions of the posterior nerve roots may result from herpes zoster, syphilis (tabes) and prolapsed intervertebral disc, but poliomyelitis affects only the anterior horn cell. Disc lesions and tumours may affect the anterior as well as the posterior nerve roots and can thus result in loss of reflexes and other motor changes as well as pain on coughing, paraesthesiae and sensory loss with ataxia.

32. (*a, b, e*)
Stereognosis (the ability to identify objects by touch) and tactile discrimination (the ability to recognize two closely placed stimuli as separate entities) are impaired by cortical lesions. The grasp reflex occurs in disorders of the frontal lobe. Dissociated anaesthesia (loss of pain and temperature sensation but retention of touch) and loss of temperature discrimination result from lesions of spinothalamic fibres.

33. (*a, c, d, e*)
Internal capsule lesions may result in contralateral hemianaesthesia, hemianopia and/or hemiplegia.

34. (*a, c, d, e*)
In syringomyelia obstruction to CSF flow causes distension of the central canal with disruption of the spinothalamic fibres as they cross the cord. The cervical cord is predominantly affected with the resulting loss of pain and temperature sensations, but retention of touch in the upper limb where there may also be wasting from involvement of the anterior horn cells. The absence of pain may lead to Charcot joints in the upper limb. Extension to the thoracic cord is marked by a level above which pain and temperature sensations are lost (suspended anaesthesia).

35. (*b, c, e*)
Tabes dorsalis is a spirochaetal infection (syphilis), which affects the dorsal column to produce ataxia and the posterior nerve roots to interrupt the afferent arc of the tendon and visceral reflexes and to cause various forms of sensory disturbance.

36. Which of the following statements about spinal cord compression are correct?

a. The spinal fluid below the lesion contains an excess of protein.
b. The sensory loss corresponds to the level of the cord lesion.
c. When root pain is present it is typically made worse by sneezing.
d. When due to trauma a spastic paraparesis or tetraparesis occurs immediately.
e. Surgery to decompress the spinal cord should never be performed within 48 hours of the development of a paraplegia.

37. The dorsal columns and corticospinal tracts are commonly affected together in

a. Syringomyelia
b. Friedreich's ataxia
c. Taboparesis
d. Tabes dorsalis
e. Subacute combined degeneration of the cord

38. Vitamin B_{12} deficiency may result in

a. Psychosis
b. Spinothalamic degeneration
c. Microcytic anaemia
d. Peripheral neuropathy
e. Ataxia

39. Friedreich's ataxia

a. Is inherited as an autosomal dominant.
b. Causes dysarthria.
c. May be accompanied by pes cavus.
d. Affects the posterior nerve roots.
e. Produces spasticity.

40. The causes of meningitis include

a. Tuberculosis
b. Viral infection
c. Osteomyelitis
d. *Haemophilus influenzae*
e. Fractured skull

Answers overleaf

36. (*a, c*)
In spinal compression the CSF below the lesion has a high protein content. Any sensory level is always two or three vertebrae lower than the actual spinal cord lesion. Root pain is typically made worse by coughing and sneezing. In sudden catastrophes (e.g. fracture of the spine) a flaccid paralysis ('spinal shock') precedes the typical spastic paraparesis or quadraparesis. If surgery is indicated, it should be performed as soon as possible to minimize permanent spinal cord damage.

37. (*b, c, e*)
Dorsal column involvement is rare and late in syringomyelia and the corticospinal tracts are never affected in tabes dorsalis.

38. (*a, d, e*)
Vitamin B_{12} deficiency results in megaloblastic macrocytic anaemia and degeneration of the corticospinal tracts and dorsal columns, the latter causing ataxia. This syndrome of subacute combined degeneration of the cord may be accompanied by psychosis and a peripheral neuropathy.

39. (*b, c, d, e*)
Friedreich's ataxia is inherited as an autosomal recessive characteristic. It affects the cerebellum to cause ataxia, nystagmus and dysarthria. Because the corticospinal tracts and posterior nerve roots are both involved, spasticity may occur in the absence of tendon reflexes. Pes cavus and scoliosis are common accompaniments of the familial neurological disorders.

40. (All correct)
Meningitis can result from infection by almost any pathogenic organism, particularly in the immunosuppressed. *Haemophilus influenzae* and (especially in the third world countries) tuberculosis are frequent causes in children, while the viruses are among the commonest causes of meningo-encephalitis in young adults. Infection with pyogenic organisms may spread to the meninges from bone sepsis around the sinuses and middle ear or after skull fracture.

41. Middle cerebral artery occlusion may cause

a. Hemianaesthesia
b. Unilateral blindness
c. Nystagmus
d. Aphasia
e. Hemiplegia

42. Conditions predisposing to stroke include

a. Atrial fibrillation
b. Myocardial infarction
c. Hypertension
d. Bacterial endocarditis
e. Diabetes

43. Vertebrobasilar insufficiency is associated with

a. Amaurosis fugax
b. Subclavian steal
c. Drop attacks
d. Cervical spondylosis
e. Vertigo

44. Subdural haemorrhage is an unlikely cause of coma if

a. There is no history of head injury.
b. Coma did not occur until several weeks after head injury.
c. There is inequality of the pupils.
d. The symptoms are fluctuant rather than progressive.
e. The patient is elderly.

45. The following are manifestations of epilepsy:

a. *Déjà vu*
b. Todd's paralysis
c. Automatism
d. Papilloedema
e. Bradykinesia

Answers overleaf

41. (*a, d, e*)
The middle cerebral artery supplies the internal capsule where infarction may result in hemianaesthesia, hemianopia, hemiplegia and (on the left side) aphasia. Unilateral blindness suggests retinal artery occlusion while nystagmus sometimes follows impairment of the vertebrobasilar circulation.

42. (All correct)
Atrial fibrillation, myocardial infarction and bacterial endocarditis may all give rise to embolism to the brain from the heart. Hypertension and diabetes predispose to atheroma with cerebral thrombosis and haemorrhage.

43. (*b, c, d, e*)
Amaurosis fugax (transient loss of vision in one eye) is usually due to microemboli in the retinal artery from an atheromatous plaque in the carotid. Vertebrobasilar insufficiency would cause hemianopia not unilateral visual loss. Occlusion of the subclavian artery proximal to the origin of the vertebral artery and also severe cervical spondylosis may both compromise the vertebral circulation.

44. (All incorrect)
These are all common features of subdural haemorrhage. Although the bleeding results from trauma to the skull, this may be so slight and so distant in time that the patient (often elderly and forgetful) cannot recall it.

45. (*a, b, c*)
Déjà vu is characteristic of temporal lobe epilepsy. Epileptic attacks may be followed by transient paralysis (Todd's paralysis) or by a period of automatism. Papilloedema is not a manifestation of epilepsy although it may accompany it when both are due to a space-occupying lesion. Bradykinesia is a feature of Parkinsonism.

46. Which of the following statements are true?

a. Symptomless hypertension does not cause stroke.
b. Convulsions in children are usually due to organic brain disease.
c. Raised intracranial pressure causes bradycardia.
d. Focal epilepsy is always idiopathic.
e. Hemianopia implies a lesion behind the optic chiasma.

47. Typical features of multiple sclerosis include

a. Cerebellar signs
b. Spastic paraplegia
c. Onset in later life
d. Progressive unremitting course
e. Diplopia

48. Cerebrospinal fluid

a. Is secreted by the arachnoid villi.
b. Pressure is raised in multiple sclerosis.
c. Sugar content is reduced in pyogenic infections.
d. Protein content may be increased in peripheral neuropathy.
e. Contains an excess of lymphocytes in viral meningitis.

49. The following are features of neurosis:

a. Interrupted sleep
b. Auditory hallucinations
c. Agoraphobia
d. Excessive sweating
e. Confabulation

50. Evidence favouring epileptic rather than hysterical attacks include

a. Nocturnal attacks
b. Resistance to passive movements
c. Lack of concern about attacks
d. Incontinence of urine
e. Regular rhythmic movements

Answers overleaf

46. (*c, e*)
Hypertension usually remains symptomless until arterial damage has already been done. Whereas convulsions may be provoked by relatively minor causes in childhood, a focal fit should always raise the possibility of a focal cerebral lesion.

47. (*a, b, e*)
Multiple sclerosis typically presents in early adult life with remissions and exacerbations. Diplopia and transient visual loss are common early symptoms, cerebellar signs are often present and many patients ultimately develop a spastic paraplegia.

48. (*c, d, e*)
The CSF is secreted from the choroid plexus and absorbed by the arachnoid villi. The pressure is normal in multiple sclerosis.

49. (*a, c, d*)
Difficulty in getting off to sleep or interrupted sleep is common in anxiety states; early morning waking is more suggestive of depression. Hallucinations and severe memory impairment with confabulation are features of a psychosis.

50. (*a, d, e*)
Hysterical attacks usually occur in the presence of witnesses and rarely in bed at night. The 'convulsive' movements are irregular and semipurposive and passive movements (e.g. attempts to force open the eyelids) are resisted. The hysterical patient displays a *belle indifference* about the attacks and rarely submits to the discomfort of urinary incontinence.

1. A 45-year-old man suddenly developed a severe headache followed by loss of consciousness. When he regained consciousness a few hours later, the headache was still present and he noticed some weakness of his left arm. Examination revealed increased tendon reflexes in the left arm and leg with an extensor plantar response on this side but no sensory changes. There were a few retinal haemorrhages but no papilloedema. No abnormality was found in the heart, lungs or abdomen. He was in sinus rhythm.

a. List the three most likely causes for this episode.
b. List the three most important modes of examination omitted from this account.

2. A 48-year-old unemployed bachelor complained of tingling in the feet, unsteadiness of gait and a poor appetite. On examination, he was unshaven and unkempt with coarse digital tremor, absent ankle jerks, impaired vibration and joint position sense in the legs, and diminished appreciation of light touch and pinprick over the feet.

a. What is the site of the neurological lesion?
b. What is the most probable cause?
c. List three abnormal signs which might be found in the abdomen.

3. List six clinical features which would favour a diagnosis of migraine in a patient presenting with headaches.

4. A 32-year-old woman complained that she was stumbling and dragging her feet after walking a short distance. She had also experienced episodes of numbness in her left arm for the past 6 months. About 7 years ago she had complained of blurred vision.

a. What is the likely diagnosis?
b. What would you expect to see in her optic fundi?
c. List three neurological signs you would expect to find in her legs.

Answers overleaf

1. *a.* (i) Subarachnoid haemorrhage
(ii) Cerebral thrombosis
(iii) Cerebral embolism
b. (i) Neck rigidity
(ii) Blood pressure
(iii) Carotid pulsation and bruits

2. *a.* Peripheral nerves in the legs
b. Alcoholic peripheral neuropathy
c. (i) Enlarged tender liver
(ii) Enlarged spleen
(iii) Ascites

3. (i) Young age of onset
(ii) Family history of migraine
(iii) Unilateral
(iv) Intermittent
(v) Preceded by transient visual or other neurological phenomena
(vi) Absence of other abnormal neurological signs

4. *a.* Multiple sclerosis
b. Pale optic discs
c. (i) Brisk reflexes
(ii) Extensor plantars
(iii) Clonus of ankles

5. A 68-year-old woman was admitted to hospital with a left hemiparesis but no impairment of light touch or pinprick sensations. She had complained of a similar episode about 1 week ago but her symptoms had resolved within 6 hours. Her pulse was irregular (120 beats/min) and the chest radiograph showed cardiomegaly with a very straight left cardiac border.

a. What is the probable cause of the hemiparesis?
b. What is the underlying diagnosis?
c. Name one likely sensory change in the affected arm.
d. What treatment must be considered?

Answers overleaf

5. *a*. Cerebral embolus
b. Mitral valve disease
c. Sensory inattention
d. Anticoagulation

Arrange the following associations into their correct pairs:

1. *A*. Dysphasia
B. Dysphonia
C. Anosmia
D. Dysarthria
E. Dyslexia

a. Larynx
b. First cranial nerve
c. Broca's area
d. Visual perception
e. Tongue

2. *A*. Raised intracranial pressure
B. Pituitary tumour
C. Middle cerebral artery thrombosis
D. Retinal artery branch embolism
E. Optic neuritis

a. Unilateral blindness
b. Homonymous hemianopia
c. Papilloedema
d. Unilateral quadrantic defect
e. Bitemporal hemianopia

3. *A*. Nystagmus
B. Bilateral ptosis
C. Constricted pupil
D. Hyperacusis
E. Positive Rinne test

a. Myasthenia gravis
b. Bell's palsy
c. Middle ear disease
d. Horner's syndrome
e. Cerebellar lesions

4. *A*. Cogwheel rigidity
B. Intention tremor
C. Fasciculation
D. Clonus
E. Myotonia

a. Cerebellum
b. Basal ganglia
c. Lower motor neurone
d. Muscle
e. Upper motor neurone

5. *A*. Romberg
B. Babinski
C. Ramsay Hunt
D. Brown-Séquard
E. Guillain–Barré

a. Posterior columns
b. Seventh cranial nerve
c. Spinal cord
d. Peripheral nerves
e. Pyramidal tract

6. *A*. Herpes zoster
B. Leprosy
C. Poliomyelitis
D. Malaria
E. *Haemophilus influenzae*

a. Cerebrum
b. Peripheral nerves
c. Meninges
d. Posterior nerve root
e. Anterior horn cell

Answers overleaf

1. *A......c*
B......a
C......b
D......e
E......d

2. *A......c*
B......e
C......b
D......d
E......a

3. *A......e*
B......a
C......d
D......b
E......c

4. *A......b*
B......a
C......c
D......e
E......d

5. *A......a*
B......e
C......b
D......c
E......d

6. *A......d*
B......b
C......e
D......a
E......c

7. *A*. Festinant
B. Scissors
C. High steppage
D. Astasia-abasia
E. Ataxic

a. Cerebellar disorders
b. Cerebral diplegia
c. Hysteria
d. Parkinsonism
e. Peripheral neuropathy

8. *A*. Spike and dome pattern
B. *Déjà vu*
C. Jacksonian
D. Clonic
E. Automatism

a. Focal convulsions
b. Post-epileptic phenomenon
c. Temporal lobe
d. Petit mal
e. Grand mal

9. *A*. Peripheral neuropathy
B. Friedreich's ataxia
C. Subacute combined
D. Tabes dorsalis
E. Multiple sclerosis

a. Demyelination
b. Spirochaetal
c. Vitamin B_{12} deficiency
d. Genetic
e. Diabetes

10. *A*. Amaurosis fugax
B. Subclavian steal
C. Hemiplegia
D. Subdural haematoma
E. Neck rigidity

a. Middle cerebral artery occlusion
b. Cerebral venous bleeding
c. Subarachnoid haemorrhage
d. Micro-emboli from carotid artery
e. Vertebral artery insufficiency

Answers overleaf

7. *A......d*
B......b
C......e
D......c
E......a

8. *A......d*
B......c
C......a
D......e
E......b

9. *A......e*
B......d
C......c
D......b
E......a

10. *A......d*
B......e
C......a
D......b
E......c

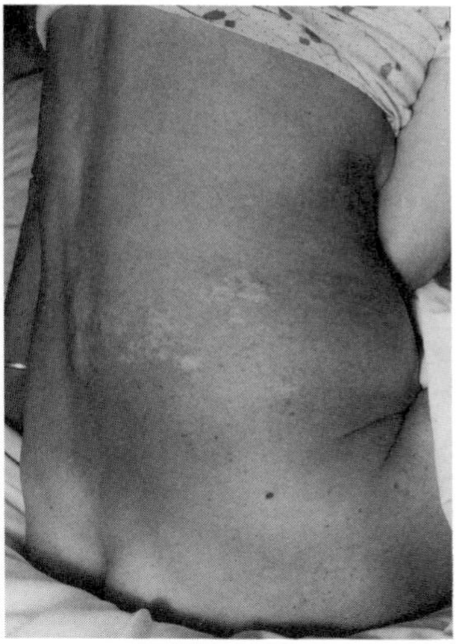

Fig. 10.1
a. From what infectious disease may this patient's grandchildren have suffered?
b. Give the exact anatomical site of the lesion causing the skin changes.

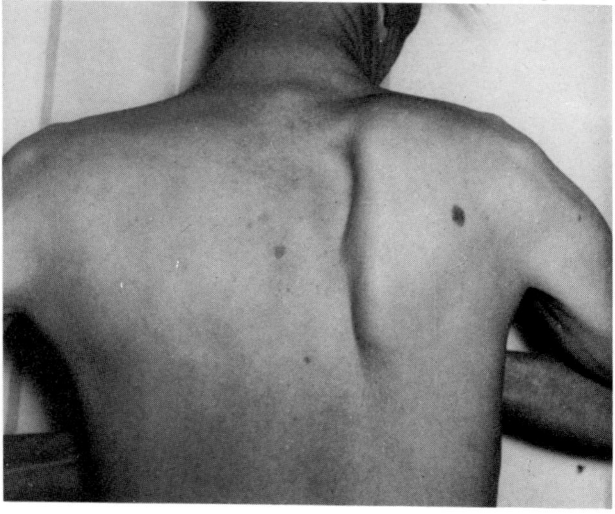

Fig. 10.2
a. What name is given to this appearance?
b. Which nerve and (or) muscle are affected?

Answers overleaf

Fig. 10.1

a. Chicken pox (the picture shows post-herpetic scarring)

b. The virus of herpes zoster mainly affects the posterior nerve roots (in this case: T10–12).

Fig. 10.2

a. Winged scapula

b. The long thoracic nerve and (or) the serratus anterior muscle

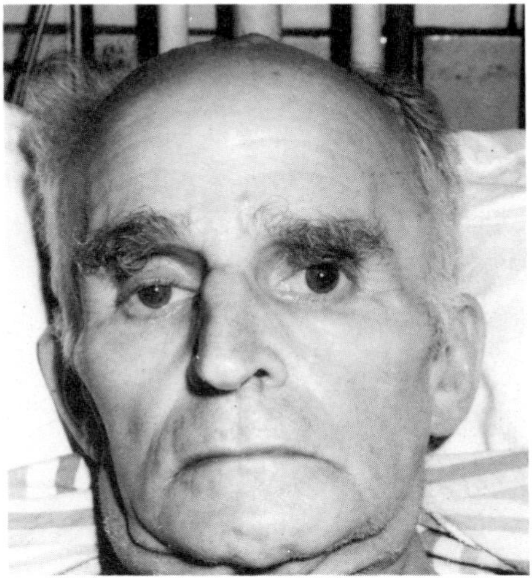

Fig. 10.3
a. What abnormality of pupil size might be found in this patient?
b. How would this help to determine the site of the causative lesion?

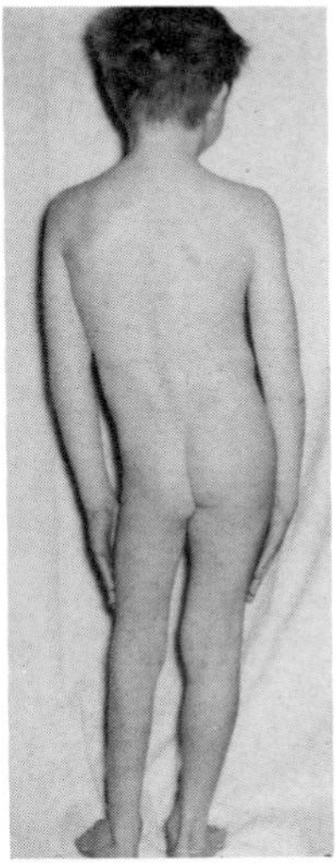

Fig. 10.4
a. List three abnormalities shown.
b. What was the most likely cause?

Answers overleaf

Fig. 10.3

a. The pupil on the side of the ptosis may be larger or smaller than the other.

b. If larger, a 3rd nerve lesion is indicated. If smaller, a lesion of the cervical sympathetic.

Fig. 10.4

a. Wasting of left leg; pelvic tilt to left and compensatory scoliosis (due to shortening of left leg).

b. Poliomyelitis

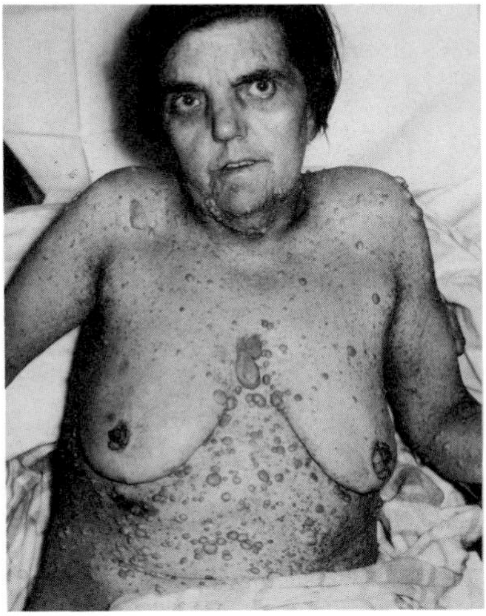

Fig. 10.5
a. What is the diagnosis?
b. Why does she have nerve deafness?

Answers overleaf

Fig. 10.5
a. Neurofibromatosis (von Recklinghausen's disease)
b. Acoustic neuroma

The Endocrine System

(Refer to Chapter 11 in *Symptoms and Signs in Clinical Medicine*, 11th edition, p. 459.)

1. A goitre may

a. Extend into the thoracic cavity.
b. Cause pulsatile jugular venous engorgement.
c. Be associated with hypothyroidism.
d. Move on swallowing.
e. Result from excessive intake of iodine.

2. Signs characteristic of pituitary tumour include

a. Loss of visual acuity
b. Optic atrophy
c. Binasal hemianopia
d. Hemiparesis
e. Anosmia

3. These conditions in childhood may cause short adult stature

a. Hyperpituitarism
b. Diabetes mellitus
c. Corticosteroid excess
d. Hypogonadism
e. Cretinism

4. Excessive loss of sodium is a characteristic feature of

a. Addison's disease
b. Cushing's syndrome
c. Diabetes insipidus
d. Hyperaldosteronism
e. Excess of vasopressin

5. Which of these are recognized features of hyperthyroidism?

a. Drowsiness
b. Pretibial myxoedema
c. Alopecia
d. Diarrhoea
e. Atrial fibrillation

Answers overleaf

1. (*a, c, d*)
An enlarged thyroid may extend behind the sternum (retrosternal goitre) and compress mediastinal structures, including the internal jugular vein or superior vena cava, to cause non-pulsatile jugular venous engorgement. A goitre may be accompanied by signs of either thyroid deficiency or excess and can result from an inadequate intake of iodine.

2. (*a, b*)
A pituitary tumour commonly involves the optic chiasma and nerves to cause bitemporal hemianopia, visual impairment and optic atrophy, and may sometimes compress the 3rd nerve, but rarely affects more distant neurological structures.

3. (*b, c, e*)
Pituitary and thyroid deficiency (cretinism) in childhood lead to short stature in adult life, whereas pituitary excess causes gigantism. Hypogonadism, by delaying puberty and epiphyseal fusion, prolongs skeletal growth. Poorly controlled diabetes or long-term treatment with corticosteroids (e.g. for asthma) tend to stunt growth.

4. (*a*)
Cushing's syndrome and hyperaldosteronism are both characterized by sodium retention due to excess of adrenal cortical hormones; in Addison's disease, there is a deficiency of these hormones. Vasopressin (the antidiuretic hormone) causes water retention; deficiency of vasopressin results in excessive loss of water rather than sodium (diabetes insipidus).

5. (*b, c, d, e*)
Drowsiness is a feature of hypothyroidism but, paradoxically, localized myxoedema especially over the shin is more common in hyperthyroidism. Hair loss (alopecia) may occur in both hyper- and hypothyroidism.

6. The eye signs of thyroid disease include

a. Suborbital swelling
b. Oculomotor pareses
c. Unequal pupils
d. Xanthelasma
e. Chemosis

7. Which of the following are neurological complications of thyroid disorder?

a. Dissociated anaesthesia
b. Carpal tunnel syndrome
c. Psychosis
d. Increased tendon reflexes with clonus
e. Diplopia

8. Which of the following statements are true of the pituitary gland?

a. Its function is regulated by the hypothalamus.
b. It lies anterior to the optic chiasma.
c. Tumours typically produce a bitemporal hemianopia.
d. ACTH is secreted by the posterior lobe.
e. Posterior lobe ablation causes fluid retention.

9. Hair loss occurs in

a. Cushing's syndrome
b. Addison's disease
c. Hyperthyroidism
d. Sheehan's syndrome
e. Conn's syndrome

10. ACTH deficiency

a. May result from post-partum haemorrhage.
b. Causes increased skin pigmentation.
c. Produces features of hypothyroidism.
d. Impairs response to stress.
e. Delays puberty.

Answers overleaf

6. (*a, b, d, e*)
Suborbital swelling from myxoedema is a typical feature of hypothyroidism and lipid deposits in the eyelids (xanthelasma) may also be seen. In hyperthyroidism, malignant ophthalmopathy may result in oedema of the conjunctiva (chemosis) and oculomotor pareses but does not affect the pupils.

7. (*b, c, e*)
Compression of the median nerve in the carpal tunnel at the wrist and delayed relaxation of tendon reflexes are found in hypothyroidism. Psychosis may complicate either hyper- or hypothyroidism. Diplopia is a symptom of malignant ophthalmopathy.

8. (*a, c*)
A pituitary tumour causes bitemporal hemianopia by compressing the crossed nasal fibres posterior to the optic chiasma. ADH (antidiuretic hormone), not ACTH, is secreted by the posterior lobe. Ablation of this lobe therefore results in polyuria.

9. (*b, c, d*)
Body hair is scanty or absent in hypopituitarism (e.g. Sheehan's syndrome). Women with decreased adrenal cortical secretion (Addison's disease) have scanty body hair, while those with excess secretion (Cushing's syndrome) are hirsute. Both hyper- and hypothyroidism may be accompanied by thinning of the head hair.

10. (*a, d*)
ACTH deficiency is part of the panhypopituitarism which results from pituitary infarction following post-partum haemorrhage. ACTH has a melanocyte-stimulating effect independent of its action upon the adrenals. Thyroid function is influenced by TSH and sexual development by GSH.

11. Diabetes mellitus is a feature of

a. Acromegaly
b. Haemochromatosis
c. Posterior pituitary ablation
d. Cushing's syndrome
e. Hyperparathyroidism

12. Osteoporosis is a characteristic finding in

a. Hypoglycaemia
b. Ovarian deficiency
c. Cushing's syndrome
d. Hypoparathyroidism
e. Hypopituitarism

13. Excessive prolactin secretion causes

a. Menorrhagia
b. Increased libido
c. Galactorrhoea
d. Hypogonadism
e. Infertility

14. Acromegaly

a. Is due to excess of growth hormone.
b. Usually presents in adolescence.
c. Causes excessive dryness of the skin.
d. Is accompanied by hypotension.
e. Leads to increase in body height.

15. Hypertension is a recognized feature of

a. Hyperthyroidism
b. Conn's syndrome
c. Adrenal medullary tumours
d. Addison's disease
e. Cushing's syndrome

Answers overleaf

11. (*a, b, d*)
Diabetes mellitus may occur with acromegaly or Cushing's syndrome and when the pancreas is damaged by iron deposition in haemochromatosis. Ablation of the posterior pituitary causes polyuria (diabetes insipidus) from deficiency of ADH.

12. (*b, c, e*)
Osteoporosis is a part of the protein-wasting effect of excessive cortisol secretion in Cushing's syndrome. Osteoporosis also results from failure of ovarian secretion as in hypopituitarism or, more commonly, following the menopause.

13. (*c, d, e*)
Increased secretion of the pituitary hormone prolactin may cause galactorrhoea but also impairs most aspects of sexual function to produce amenorrhoea, loss of libido, hypogonadism and infertility.

14. (*a*)
Acromegaly is due to excess of growth hormone arising in adult life after the epiphyses have fused. It thus causes thickening but not lengthening of the bones. Increased height (gigantism) occurs only if there is excess of growth hormone before epiphyseal fusion. Moist greasy skin and hypertension are other features of the disease.

15. (*b, c, e*)
Hypertension may result from excessive secretion of aldosterone (Conn's syndrome), cortisol (Cushing's syndrome) or catecholamines (phaeochromocytoma of the adrenal medulla). Hyperthyroidism may cause a large pulse volume but not true hypertension. Addison's disease is characterized by hypotension.

16. Autoimmunity is an acknowledged cause of

a. Hypothyroidism
b. Addison's disease
c. Cushing's syndrome
d. Hyperthyroidism
e. Hyperparathyroidism

17. Gynaecomastia is associated with

a. Klinefelter's syndrome
b. Turner's syndrome
c. Hepatic cirrhosis
d. Spironolactone therapy
e. Bronchial carcinoma

18. Convulsions are a recognized characteristic of

a. Turner's syndrome
b. Islet-cell tumour of pancreas
c. Hypoparathyroidism
d. Klinefelter's syndrome
e. Inappropriate secretion of ADH

19. Ocular signs of parathyroid disease include:

a. Blepharospasm
b. Ptosis
c. Corneal calcification
d. Cataract
e. Arcus senilis

20. Diabetes mellitus

a. Can present in childhood or old age.
b. May be associated with hyperlipidaemia.
c. Predisposes to pyelonephritis.
d. Causes proximal muscle wasting.
e. May be due to haemochromatosis.

Answers overleaf

16. (*a, b, d*)
Autoimmunity is an important cause of endocrine hypofunction, and especially of hypothyroidism, hypoparathyroidism and Addison's disease, but it is also responsible for some cases of hyperthyroidism (Graves' disease). Cushing's syndrome and hyperparathyroidism are examples of excessive endocrine secretion due to hyperplasia or tumour of the secreting cells.

17. (*a, c, d, e*)
Gynaecomastia is a feature of Klinefelter's syndrome, a genetic abnormality in men, but Turner's syndrome in women is characterized by poorly developed breasts with widely spaced nipples. The failure by a damaged liver to detoxicate oestrogens is another cause of gynaecomastia. Certain drugs can produce gynaecomastia, including spironolactone and digoxin.

18. (*b, c, e*)
The causes of convulsions of endocrine origin include hypoglycaemia, hypocalcaemia and cerebral oedema due to excessive production of antidiuretic hormone. Rarely, tumours of the pituitary may by their local effects produce convulsions as may hypertensive crises in patients with endocrine causes for a raised blood pressure (e.g. phaeochromocytoma).

19. (*a, c, d*)
Hypocalcaemia due to hypoparathyroidism may cause muscle twitching, including blepharospasm (twitching of eyelids), and also cataract. The hypercalcaemia of hyperparathyroidism can lead to deposition of calcium in the cornea. This can be distinguished by its site from the lipid deposition of arcus senilis.

20. (All correct)
Diabetes may present acutely in early life when it is usually responsive to insulin or more insidiously in later life when it is usually insulin resistant. It may rarely be due to deposition of iron in the pancreas (haemochromatosis). The complications include arterial disease due to hyperlipidaemia, infection, such as pyelonephritis, peripheral neuropathy and proximal myopathy.

1. A 35-year-old woman presented with a 6-month history of amenorrhoea, diarrhoea, weight loss and palpitations. She had also been having serious marital difficulties and had been seen by a psychiatrist, who diagnosed an acute anxiety state and prescribed a tranquillizer but without any benefit.

a. What is the most important organic disease to exclude?

b. List five abnormal signs which would support this diagnosis.

2. A 60-year-old man was admitted to hospital in a coma which had been preceded by convulsions. He recovered consciousness overnight without any residual neurological signs and was able to take fluids normally. He was then able to give a 2-month history of cough, sputum, haemoptysis and weight loss. Later that day, he again lapsed into a coma from which he spontaneously aroused some hours later. Examination of the blood showed abnormally low values for serum urea and electrolytes.

a. Give two possible causes for the convulsions and coma.

b. What is the most likely cause of the respiratory symptoms?

Answers overleaf

1. *a*. Hyperthyroidism
b. (i) Digital tremor
(ii) Hot, moist skin
(iii) Tachycardia
(iv) Goitre with overlying bruit
(v) Eye signs: exophthalmos, lid-lag, etc.

2. *a*. (i) Inappropriate secretion of ADH
(ii) Cerebral metastases
b. Small-cell carcinoma of the bronchus

Arrange the following associations into their correct pairs:

1. *A*. Long limbs
   B. Truncal obesity
   C. Enlarged distal parts
   D. Dwarfism
   E. Gigantism

   a. Acromegaly
   b. Prepubertal hyperpituitarism
   c. Eunuchoidism
   d. Cushing's syndrome
   e. Prepubertal hypopituitarism

2. *A*. Fragile skin
   B. Pigmented skin
   C. Hot moist skin
   D. Xanthelasma
   E. Absent body hair

   a. Addison's disease
   b. Hyperthyroidism
   c. Cushing's syndrome
   d. Sheehan's syndrome
   e. Diabetes

3. *A*. Tetany
   B. Hypertension
   C. Hypotension
   D. Polyuria
   E. Bitemporal hemianopia

   a. Hyperparathyroidism
   b. Hypoparathyroidism
   c. Pituitary tumour
   d. Phaeochromocytoma
   e. Waterhouse–Friderichsen syndrome

4. *A*. Low serum sodium
   B. High ACTH
   C. Increased T3
   D. Low serum calcium
   E. Increased hydroxycorticosteroids

   a. Cataract
   b. Pigmentation
   c. Osteoporosis
   d. Tachycardia
   e. Hypotension

5. *A*. Decreased serum osmolality
   B. Delayed relaxation of tendon reflexes
   C. Positive Chvostek's sign
   D. Pretibial myxoedema
   E. Peripheral neuropathy

   a. Hypoparathyroidism
   b. Hypothyroidism
   c. Inappropriate ADH secretion
   d. Diabetes mellitus
   e. Hyperthyroidism

Answers overleaf

1. *A......c*
B......d
C......a
D......e
E......b

2. *A......c*
B......a
C......b
D......e
E......d

3. *A......b*
B......d
C......e
D......a
E......c

4. *A......e*
B......b
C......d
D......a
E......c

5. *A......c*
B......b
C......a
D......e
E......d

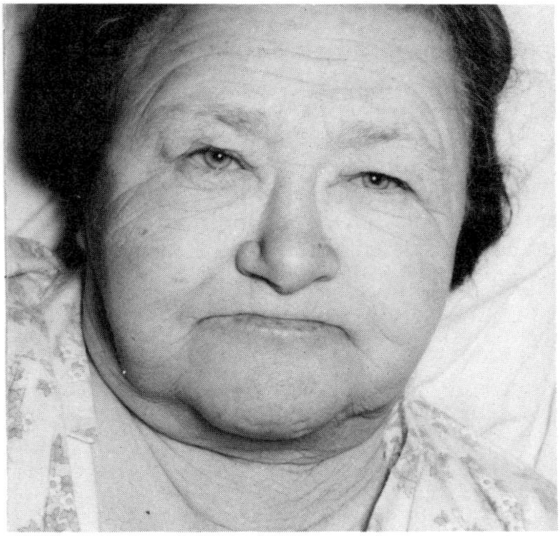

Fig. 11.1
a. Give three symptoms of which this patient might complain.
b. What reflex abnormality might be found?

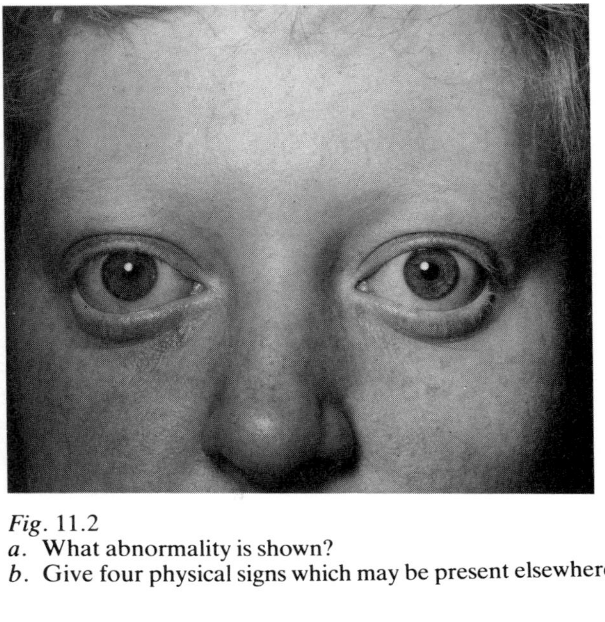

Fig. 11.2
a. What abnormality is shown?
b. Give four physical signs which may be present elsewhere.

Answers overleaf

Fig. 11.1

a. Fatigue; 'slowing up'; constipation; feeling the cold; deafness; hoarse voice.

b. Delayed relaxation of tendon reflexes

Fig. 11.2

a. Exophthalmos (rin of sclera visible between iris and lower lid)

b. Goitre with overlying bruit; hot moist skin; digital tremor; tachycardia

Tropical Diseases

(Refer to Chapter 12 in *Symptoms and Signs in Clinical Medicine*, 11th edition, p. 483.)

1. Which of the following typical associations with fever are correct?

a. Continuous fever and initial attack of tertian malaria
b. Double diurnal temperature rise and *Borrelia* genus infections
c. 'Saddleback' temperature and kala-azar
d. Rigors and falling temperature
e. High temperature with relatively slow pulse and Chagas' disease

2. Skin manifestations of specific tropical diseases include:

a. Increased melanin in patients suffering from kala-azar
b. Diminished pigmentation in yaws
c. Circinate rash with dengue infections
d. Macular lesions in leprosy
e. Creeping cutaneous eruptions with nematode larvae infections

3. Recognized features of infective tropical diarrhoeas are:

a. Colonic bleeding
b. Severe muscle cramps
c. Trismus
d. Malabsorption
e. 'Rice-water' stools

4. Which of the following physical signs are recognized features of the disease listed in brackets?

a. Black discoloration of the tongue (riboflavin deficiency)
b. Magenta tongue (tropical sprue)
c. Koplik spots (measles)
d. Painless enlargement of the parotid (malnutrition)
e. Extreme dryness of the tongue (Ebola virus infection)

5. Tender hepatomegaly is a characteristic feature of

a. Amoebic abscess
b. Brucellosis
c. Leprosy
d. Hydatid disease
e. Malaria

Answers overleaf

1. (*a*)
Fever in tropical disease is usually associated with a tachycardia, although in yellow fever the pulse is often disproportionately slow (the opposite being the case in Chagas' disease). Rigors classically occur when the temperature rises rapidly. The classic fever of tertian and quartan malaria is not usually seen in the initial illness. Kala-azar (not *Borrelia* genus infections) causes double diurnal temperature rise, and dengue is characterized by a saddleback temperature curve.

2. (*a, b, d, e*)
A wide variety of rashes are seen in tropical diseases. There is an increase in melanin ('black sickness') in kala-azar and a decrease in pigmentation in yaws. The macular rash in leprosy is also associated with hypopigmentation. Dengue results in bright red macules and African trypanosomiasis in a circinate rash. Nematode larvae are characterized by a creeping cutaneous eruption.

3. (*a, b, d, e*)
Colonic bleeding, muscle cramps due to electrolyte loss, tenesmus (trismus is painful spasm of the jaw muscles), malabsorption and 'rice-water' stools (in cholera) are all features found in tropical diarrhoeas.

4. (*c, d, e*)
A smooth red tongue is typical of tropical sprue and magenta coloration is seen in riboflavin deficiency. A black discoloration is due to fungal colonization.

5. (*a, b, e*)
All these diseases result in hepatomegaly, but it is not characteristically tender in leprosy and hydatid disease.

6. Splenomegaly may be found in

a. Trypanosomiasis
b. Leptospirosis
c. Thalassaemia
d. Typhus fever
e. Visceral leishmaniasis

7. Which of the following diseases can directly damage the heart and/or pericardium?

a. Leprosy
b. *Trypanosoma rhodesiense*
c. Amoebiasis
d. Chagas' disease
e. Leptospirosis

8. Which of the following are recognized respiratory complications of the stated disease?

a. Inflammation at the right lung base in patients with hepatic amoebiasis
b. Pulmonary oedema with falciparum malaria
c. Katayama syndrome (cough, fever, urticaria and eosinophilia) with yellow fever
d. Pleural effusion and African trypanosomiasis
e. Haemoptysis with paragonamiasis

9. The renal manifestations of *Schistosoma haematobium* include

a. Hydronephrosis
b. Cystitis
c. Chyluria
d. Haemoglobinuria
e. Bladder polypi

10. Which of the following are characteristic neurological complications?

a. Convulsions associated with *Plasmodium vivax* malaria
b. Enlarged tender peripheral nerves in patients with kuru
c. Delirium and coma associated with African trypanosomiasis
d. Foot drop due to thiamine deficiency
e. Neuropathic joint injury due to leprosy

Answers overleaf

6. (All correct)
Splenomegaly is a feature of a large number of tropical diseases including all those mentioned.

7. (*b, c, d, e*)
Chagas' disease (due to *Trypanosoma cruzi*) may produce a severe myocarditis in children and this has also been reported in African trypanosomiasis. Other causes of myocarditis include toxoplasmosis, trichinosis and leptospirosis. Amoebiasis and scrub typhus are causes of pericarditis.

8. (*a, b, d, e*)
A patient suffering from hepatic amoebiasis frequently complains of right pleuritic and shoulder-tip pain. The chest radiograph typically reveals an elevated right hemidiaphragm and inflammatory shadowing sometimes with effusion. Katayama syndrome is associated with the invasive stage of *Schistosoma mansoni* infections. Tropical 'eosinophilic lung' is most commonly due to filarial worms of animal origin. African trypanosomiasis may be complicated by a pleural effusion.

9. (*a, b, e*)
The renal manifestations of *Schistosoma haematobium* include cystitis, haematuria (not haemoglobinuria), bladder ulceration and polypi. Sometimes the ureters become stenosed and this then results in hydronephrosis. Chyluria is due to obstruction of the abdominal lymphatics in filariasis.

10. (*c, d, e*)
Convulsions occur with falciparum malaria but are not characteristic of *Plasmodium vivax*. Enlarged, tender palpable nerves and neuropathic joints are features of leprosy. Thiamine deficiency is a cause of peripheral neuropathy which can result in wrist and foot drop. Delirium can occur with any high fever but is especially common in falciparum malaria, African trypanosomiasis and Japanese B encephalitis.

11. The diseases listed are typically associated with the following ocular complications:

a. Trachoma with conjunctival follicles
b. Riboflavin deficiency with keratomalacia
c. Leptospirosis with subconjunctival haemorrhages
d. Leprosy with paralytic lagophthalmos
e. Loiasis with 'snow-flake' opacities

12. The organisms causing the following diseases are found in the blood using simple light microscopy:

a. Typhus
b. Trypanosomiasis
c. Yellow fever
d. Ancylostomiasis
e. Malaria due to *Plasmodium ovale*

13. Blood eosinophilia is typical of the following infections:

a. Filariasis
b. Loiasis
c. Cholera
d. *Ascaris lumbricoides*
e. Brucellosis

14. Which of the following statements about blood films are correct?

a. A wet preparation is most useful for demonstrating motile bacteria.
b. Thick films are the best way of diagnosing malaria.
c. Trypanosomes can be adequately diagnosed on thin films.
d. When looking for microfilariae the blood should be taken between 6 and 10 a.m.
e. Thick films are typically stained with Leishman's stain.

15. Which of the organisms causing the following diseases are typically found in faeces?

a. Amoebiasis
b. Schistosomiasis (due to *Schistosoma mansoni*)
c. Trachoma
d. Hydatid disease
e. Kala-azar

Answers overleaf

11. (*a, c, d*)
Ocular problems are a common manifestation of tropical diseases. Trachoma is characterized by follicles on the palpebral conjunctiva. Riboflavin deficiency can result in vascularization of the sclera and vitamin A deficiency in dryness of the eye and keratomalacia. Leprosy can result in inability to close the eyes (lagophthalmos) that leads to severe corneal damage and even perforation. 'Snow-flake' opacities are a feature of onchocerciasis (not loiasis) and leptospirosis is a cause of subconjunctival haemorrhages.

12. (*b, e*)
Yellow fever is caused by a virus and typhus by a rickettsia, neither of which can be seen with normal light microscopy. Ancylostomiasis is hook-worm infestation of the bowel.

13. (*a, b, d*)
Blood eosinophilia is particularly common in helminthic infections. It is not typical of cholera or brucellosis.

14. (*b, c*)
A wet preparation is used to demonstrate motile protozoa not bacteria. Thick films (prepared with Giemsa's or Field's stain) are the classic way to diagnose malaria; other parasites such as trypanosomes can equally well be seen on thin films. Nocturnal microfilariae are seen in the blood between 10 p.m. and 2 a.m. and diurnal microfilariae around midday.

15. (*a, b*)
Amoebiasis and schistosomiasis organisms are found in the stool. *Echinococcus granulosus* (the cause of hydatid disease), although gaining entry via the gastrointestinal tract, is not retrieved from the stools.

1. Twenty days after returning from West Africa a 35-year-old business executive developed a continuous fever, muscle and joint pains and headaches. He had tender hepatosplenomegaly. His blood count showed a mild leucopenia and anaemia.

a. What is the most important diagnosis to exclude?
b. List four recognized complications of this condition.
c. How would you confirm the diagnosis?

2. A man who travelled widely in tropical countries developed fever, drenching sweats, upper right abdominal and lower chest pain. On examination, he was found to have tender hepatomegaly and reduced percussion note at the right lung base with bronchial breathing. The chest radiograph showed a high right diaphragm and an overlying effusion.

a. What is the most likely diagnosis?
b. What is the causative organism?
c. Name the two commonest modes of transmission.

Answers overleaf

1. *a*. Malignant tertian malaria (*Plasmodium falciparum*)
b. (i) Neurological complications (delirium, convulsions, coma)
(ii) Renal insufficiency
(iii) Haemolytic anaemia
(iv) Haemoglobinuria
(v) Hyperpyrexia
(vi) Algid malaria (producing a shock syndrome)
c. Thick blood film

2. *a*. Amoebic liver abscess
b. *Entamoeba histolytica*
c. (i) Food
(ii) Water supplies

Arrange the following associations into their correct pairs:

1. *A*. 'Saddleback' fever — *a*. Measles
B. Diminished pigmentation — *b*. African trypanosomiasis
C. Circinate rash — *c*. Leprosy
D. Creeping cutaneous eruption — *d*. Nematode infection
E. Koplic spots — *e*. Dengue

2. *A*. 'Rice-water' stools — *a*. Measles
B. Magenta tongue — *b*. Cholera
C. Koplik spots — *c*. Riboflavin deficiency
D. Tender hepatomegaly — *d*. Leprosy
E. Painless splenomegaly — *e*. Hydatid disease

3. *A*. Myocarditis — *a*. *Schistosoma haematobium*
B. Pleural effusion — *b*. Filariasis
C. Haematuria — *c*. Leprosy
D. Chyluria — *d*. African trypanosomiasis
E. Tender peripheral nerves — *e*. Chagas' disease

4. *A*. Conjunctival follicles — *a*. Thiamine deficiency
B. Subconjunctival haemorrhages — *b*. Filariasis
C. Gross blood eosinophilia — *c*. Schistosomiasis
D. Foot drop — *d*. Trachoma
E. Bladder polypi — *e*. Leptospirosis

Answers overleaf

1. *A......e*
B......c
C......b
D......d
E......a

2. *A......b*
B......c
C......a
D......e
E......d

3. *A......e*
B......d
C......a
D......b
E......c

4. *A......d*
B......e
C......b
D......a
E......c

The Examination of Children

(Refer to Chapter 13 in *Symptoms and Signs in Clinical Medicine*, 11th edition, p. 500.)

1. Which of the following observations are used to assess the Apgar score in a newborn infant?

a. Colour
b. Pupillary reflex
c. Reflex irritability
d. Heart rate
e. Blood pressure

2. Which of the following statements about the inspection of a newborn infant are correct?

a. The 'frog' position is typical of the full-term infant.
b. Body odour may suggest inborn errors of metabolism.
c. Erythema toxicum is due to streptococcal skin infection.
d. Mongolian blue spots are due to birth trauma.
e. Capillary haemangiomas on the eyelids are typically of no clinical significance.

3. Neonatal jaundice

a. Which occurs within the first 24 hours is typically 'physiological'.
b. Is a complication of galactosaemia.
c. When prolonged is a feature of congenital hypothyroidism.
d. Is a cause of deafness.
e. When due to 'neonatal hepatitis' is caused by maternal alcoholism.

4. Cyanosis in the newborn is associated with the following:

a. Diaphragmatic hernia
b. Meningitis
c. Patent foramen ovale
d. Choanal atresia
e. Hypoglycaemia

Answers overleaf

1. (*a, c, d*)
The Apgar score reflects the infant's general condition 1 and 5 min after delivery and depends on colour, heart rate, respiration, reflex irritability and muscle tone.

2. (*b, e*)
The 'frog' position (widely abducted thighs and flexed knees when lying supine) results from hypotonia and weakness and is characteristic of the pre-term infant. Body odours occasionally help in diagnosing metabolic disorders. Erythema toxicum is common, has no clinical significance but must be distinguished from staphlococcal lesions. Mongolian blue spots occur when one or both parents are coloured and are of no clinical significance.

3. (*b, c, d*)
Jaundice appearing within 24 hours is usually pathological (galactosaemia being a rare cause). Physiological jaundice tends to occur later and, if prolonged, may indicate hypothyroidism. Neonatal jaundice particularly in the premature is a cause of perceptive deafness.

4. (*a, b, d, e*)
Respiratory distress is caused by a large number of conditions, including all those listed apart from patent foramen ovale which, if isolated, is of little clinical significance.

5. Which of the following statements about the head and facies are correct:

a. High-set ears are a marker of congenital defects.
b. The edge of a cephalhaematoma often calcifies.
c. A closed posterior fontanelle at birth is associated with mental retardation.
d. Dimples in the nape of the neck are associated with central nervous system abnormalities.
e. Caput succedaneum is associated with anaemia.

6. Which of the following findings when examining the chest and heart are always abnormal?

a. Respiratory rate of more than 30/min
b. Grunting respiration
c. Systolic murmurs
d. Heart rate of 160 beats/min
e. Sternal recession

7. Which of the following findings on abdominal and genital examination are always abnormal?

a. Two umbilical arteries
b. A palpable liver
c. A trace of blood from the vagina
d. Palpable kidneys
e. Prominent labia minora

8. Which of the following statements about the limbs and back are correct?

a. A sinus anywhere above the S2 segment should be surgically excised.
b. Supernumerary digits are typically associated with an encephalocoele.
c. Subluxation of the hips cannot be treated until an infant is 6 months old.
d. Talipes is an abnormality of the hands.
e. A hairy patch over the lower back is of no significance.

Answers overleaf

5. (*b, d*)
Low-, not high-, set ears are associated with congenital defects. A cephalhaematoma may produce anaemia soon after birth and later resolve, leaving a calcified edge. Caput succedaneum does not produce anaemia, being scalp oedema after birth. A closed posterior fossa at birth is common and of no significance. Dimples in posterior midline may communicate with the central nervous system.

6. (*b*)
In the newborn the respiratory rate may be up to 40/min and the heart rate up to 180 beats/min. Systolic murmurs are common and often of no significance and similarly some degree of sternal recession is frequently seen. However, grunting respiration is always abnormal.

7. (All correct)
All these findings may be present in the newborn. The trace of blood from the vagina is due to maternal oestrogen withdrawal.

8. (*a*)
Any sinus above the S2 segment may communicate with the theca and requires surgical removal. Subluxation of the hips requires treatment very soon after birth (hips kept in abduction) and talipes is a deformity of the feet (club foot). Polydactyly runs in families, being particularly common in Africans, and is not typically associated with an encephalocoele. Spina bifida occulta may be marked by a tuft of hair on the lower back.

9. Convulsions in the newborn

a. Are rarely generalized.
b. Are associated with milia neonatorum.
c. May be due to hypocalcaemia.
d. Are associated with milia neonatorum.
e. Should lead to immediate measurement of the blood sugar.

10. The Moro reflex

a. Is abnormal after 6 months of age.
b. Is elicited by rapidly elevating an infant's head.
c. Should be performed when the infant is asleep.
d. If asymmetrical, suggests birth injury.
e. If exaggerated, may be due to a metabolic disturbance.

11. Which of the following statements about the primitive reflexes are correct?

a. Rooting reflex is normal until the age of 12 months.
b. Sucking reflex is elicited by stroking the infant's cheek.
c. Plantar grasp reflex can override a positive Babinski's sign.
d. The asymmetrical tense neck reflex produces flexion of the ipsilateral arm and extension of the contralateral leg.
e. The palmar grasp reflex is normally present for the first 3–4 months of life.

12. A small-for-dates baby

a. Has a birth weight more than 2 standard deviations below the mean weight for gestational age.
b. May be caused by intra-uterine cytomegalovirus infection.
c. May have its gestation age accurately assessed by using the criteria described by Dubowitz.
d. Is associated with maternal rubella.
e. Is more liable to meconium aspiration.

13. A premature baby is typically predisposed to the following complications:

a. Intraventricular haemorrhage
b. Polycythaemia
c. Hyaline membrane disease
d. Necrotizing enterocolitis
e. Hypoglycaemia

Answers overleaf

9. (*a, c, e*)
Convulsions in the neonate are more often focal than generalized and are most frequently due to birth. Other causes include congenital malformations and are most frequently due to birth or to metabolic disturbances such as hypoglycaemia (hence the importance of measuring the blood sugar) or hypocalcaemia. Milia neonatorum are white pinhead lesions over the nose and are very common in normal babies.

10. (*a, d, e*)
The Moro reflex is always abnormal after 6 months of age, is elicited by allowing the head to fall a few centimetres and is best performed with the infant wide awake. Birth injury can produce both an asymmetrical and/or exaggerated response. Metabolic disturbances also produce exaggeration of the reflex.

11. (*c, e*)
The rooting reflex elicited by stroking the infant's cheek is present up to 4 months of age as is the palmar grasp reflex. The asymmetrical tense neck reflex produces extension of the ipsilateral arm and flexion of the contralateral leg. Care must always be taken not to overlook a positive Babinski's sign in the presence of a grasp reflex.

12. (All correct)
The birth weight of a small-for-dates baby is more than 2 standard deviations below the mean weight for gestational age and may be due to maternal infection such as cytomegalovirus and rubella. The Dubowitz criteria allow determination of gestational age to within ±2 weeks. Meconium aspiration, polycythaemia and hypoglycaemia are problems encountered with such babies.

13. (*a, c, d, e*)
All these problems with the exception of polycythaemia are typically encountered with prematurity.

14. Which of the following physical features are useful in assessing gestational age?

a. Nipple formation
b. Oedema
c. Ear firmness
d. Plantar creases
e. Skin opacity

15. Examination of the hip joints

a. Is best performed at the beginning of a clinical examination.
b. Should be with the hips slightly flexed (approx 20°).
c. A clicking sound is associated with congenital dislocation.
d. Barlow's manoeuvre is used to elicit hip instability.
e. Minor degrees of hip instability are best elicited with the infant in the prone position.

16. Which of the following milestones in development should have occurred by the times indicated?

a. Able to sit unsupported at 6 months.
b. Smiles at mother at 4 to 6 weeks.
c. Reaches for an object at 8 weeks.
d. Helps with dressing by holding out appropriate arm or foot at 10 months.
e. Uses two or three words with meaning at 8 months.

17. Which of the following statements about development are correct?

a. Emotional deprivation may result in delayed milestones.
b. Sitting and walking are the best overall guide to development.
c. Prematurity does not influence development after 4 weeks of age.
d. A specific handicap should be considered if there is a marked delay in a single milestone.
e. Prolonged hospitalization is a recognized cause of marked delay in milestones.

Answers overleaf

14. (All correct)
In all, Dubowitz described eleven external signs useful in determining gestational age.

15. (*c, d*)
For examination, the infant lies supine the hips being flexed at right-angle with the knees fully flexed. A clicking sound associated with a 'jerk' is produced by the head of the femur slipping into the acetabulum. Barlow's manoeuvre does elicit hip instability. The hips are best left to the end of the clinical examination as the child usually resents the procedure.

16. (*b, d*)
A normal baby smiles at mother by 6 weeks, reaches for an object by 5 months, sits unaided by 8 months, helps with dressing by 10 months and uses three or four words with meaning by the end of the first year.

17. (*a, d, e*)
Milestones may be delayed in an otherwise normal child due to emotional deprivation, prematurity or prolonged hospitalization. Delay in all the milestones is much more significant than delay in sitting and walking, both of which are subject to wide variations. Marked delay in a single milestone may be due to a specific handicap (e.g. speech and deafness).

18. Pathologically abnormal facies are commonly associated with

a. Finger-like thumbs
b. Overlapping fingers
c. Abnormally long fingers
d. Proximally placed thumbs
e. Unusual palmar crease patterns

19. Which of the following are recognized features of hypothyroidism in infants?

a. Macroglossia
b. Bulky muscles
c. Defective dentition
d. Diarrhoea
e. Umbilical hernia

20. Turner's syndrome is associated with

a. Puffiness of the hands
b. Multiple naevi
c. Delayed femoral pulses
d. Sparse hair
e. Hoarse cry

21. Which of the following statements about the skull are correct?

a. Bossing of the skull is a feature of thalassaemia.
b. Hydranencephaly is associated with marked transillumination.
c. Craniotabes is a finding in oxycephaly.
d. 'Cracked pot' note on percussing the skull is typical of raised intracranial pressure.
e. Hydrocephalus is associated with a rapidly increasing head circumference.

22. Dehydration

a. First produces clinical signs when fluid loss is 30 per cent of body weight.
b. With a rubbery feel to the skin suggests hyernatraemia.
c. Is a recognized complication of fluid exudate in the small bowel without diarrhoea.
d. Characteristically causes a sunken fontanelle.
e. When isotonic typically results in irritability.

Answers overleaf

18. (All correct)
Abnormal facies are associated with many congenital disorders including all those listed.

19. (*a, b, c, e*)
The clinical features of hypothyroidism (which develop over many months) include pallor, dry skin, puffy eyes, macroglossia, bulky muscles, poor dentition, growth retardation and constipation (not diarrhoea).

20. (*a, b, c*)
Turner's syndrome (ovarian dysgenesis) is due to chromosome abnormalities and is characterized by short stature, webbing of the neck, puffiness of hands, naevi and a low-set posterior hair line. Coarctation is the commonest associated cardiac defect (hence delayed femoral pulses).

21. (*a, b, d, e*)
Bossing of the skull is characteristic of rickets and chronic haemolytic anaemias such as thalassaemia. Hydranencephaly (where most of the cerebrum is destroyed leaving a thin membrane enclosing the ventricles) and to a lesser degree hydrocephalus are associated with increased transillumination. In both these conditions the head circumference rapidly increases in size. Craniotabes occurs when the skull bones are soft (e.g. rickets).

22. (*b, c, d*)
Signs of dehydration occur when the fluid loss is 5–10 per cent of total body mass. The fontanelle becomes sunken, skin turgor is lost and, in the presence of hypernatraemia, the skin may have a rubbery feel. Dehydration may be apparent before the onset of diarrhoea if large quantities of fluid are sequestered in the small bowel. Isotonic dehydration usually results in lethargy.

23. Which of the following statements about precordial thrills felt in infancy are correct?

a. The thrill associated with a ventricular septal defect is typically maximal at the left sternal edge.
b. It is recognized that thrills may radiate to the epigastriun.
c. Vibrations arising in the airways are easily confused with a cardiac thrill.
d. Thrills are easy to localize in children because of their thin chest walls.
e. Small atrial septal defects classically produce a marked thrill at the apex.

24. Which of the following statements about murmurs and heart sounds are correct?

a. Innocent murmurs fluctuate in intensity.
b. Venous hum is accentuated by gentle compression of the jugular vein.
c. Murmur of patent ductus arteriosus is best heard below the right clavicle.
d. Splitting of the pulmonary second sound is always pathological in children.
e. Functional murmurs classically increase in intensity on inspiration.

25. When examining the central nervous system in infants

a. Fanning of the fingers on reaching for an object is characteristic of spasticity.
b. Neuromuscular disease typically results in growth retardation of the affected limb.
c. Hypotonic infants can never hold their limbs against gravity.
d. A Babinski reflex overrides a persistent plantar grasp reflex.
e. Manipulation of building blocks is a poor method of assessing fine movement of the hands.

Answers overleaf

23. (*a, b, c*)
In infants thrills arising from the heart radiate widely throughout the precordium (occasionally into the epigastrium) and are thus difficult to localize. Occasionally they can be easily confused with vibrations arising in the airways. A ventricular septal defect classically results in a thrill maximal at the left sternal edge, while a small atrial septal defect does not produce a thrill.

24. (*a*)
Innocent murmurs are 'ejection' systolic, soft, tend to decrease in intensity in the erect posture and on inspiration. Venous hum always disappears on gentle compression of the jugular veins. The murmur of patent ductus arteriosus is often best heard below the left, not right, clavicle, and splitting of the pulmonary second sound is common in normal children.

25. (*a, b*)
Manipulation of wooden blocks is a good test of both cortico-visio-spatial perception and fine movements of the hands. With a spastic upper limb such manipulation is poor and, in addition, there is fanning of the fingers and external rotation. Neuromuscular disease often results in growth retardation, and hypotonic infants without weakness can hold their limbs against gravity.

26. Which of the following statements about examination of the ears in infants are correct?

a. Examination should never be attempted with the child restrained.
b. The tympanic membrane is normally grey and translucent.
c. Serous otitis media results in loss of the light reflex.
d. Hearing deficiency is easily demonstrated clinically by 9 months of age.
e. The auditory canal in infants is characteristically tortuous.

27. Ulceration of the mouth and lips

a. Is caused by herpes simplex.
b. Is a feature of severe monilial infections.
c. Is a typical finding in scurvy.
d. In children is very frequently associated with fever.
e. Is a recognized presenting feature of acute leukaemia.

28. Which of the following statements about the mouth are correct?

a. Use of tetracycline in early childhood results in an increased incidence of dental caries.
b. Koplik's spots are pathognomonic of rubella.
c. Petechiae on the palate are a feature of herpangina.
d. The tonsillar pseudomembrane due to infectious mononucleosis is easily wiped off the tonsils.
e. Bright orange tonsils are associated with Tangier disease.

29. Stridor

a. Is usually trivial when due to epiglottitis.
b. Secondary to retropharyngeal abscess typically results in flexion of the neck.
c. Is a symptom of inhalation of a foreign body.
d. Is associated with hypocalcaemia.
e. Should always lead to immediate and thorough examination of the throat.

Answers overleaf

26. (*b, c*)
When examining the ears a child must always be held firmly. The auditory canal is straight (unlike adults) and the drum grey and translucent. Loss of the light reflex is common in middle-ear disease. Hearing deficiency can be extraordinarily difficult to demonstrate in young children.

27. (*a, d, e*)
The commonest cause of mouth ulceration is herpes simplex infection and this may be associated with constitutional upset. Ulceration is not a feature of monilial infections or scurvy but is common in acute leukaemias.

28. (*a, c, d, e*)
Tetracycline should not be prescribed in pregnancy or early childhood because the teeth may be discoloured and have defective enamel. Koplik's spots are pathognomonic of measles (not German measles). Petechiae on the palate are commonly seen with infectious mononucleosis and herpangina. In contrast to diphtheria, the exudate in infectious mononucleosis is less easily scraped off. Bright orange tonsils are seen in the very rare condition Tangier disease.

29. (*c, d*)
Epiglottitis is one of the most serious causes of stridor in a child as it may result in complete airway obstruction, particularly after examination of the throat. Retropharyngeal abscess typically results in extension of the neck.

30. Which of the following facts about pubertal development are correct?

a. Breast enlargement in adolescent boys is invariably pathological.
b. Testicular volume increases before other signs of puberty.
c. The average age for the onset of menstruation is 11·8 years.
d. Breast development is the first sign of puberty in girls.
e. Testicular development is measured by the Prader orchidometer.

Answers overleaf

30. (*b, d, e*)
The earliest signs of puberty in boys is increase in testicular volume (measured by a Prader orchidometer) and in girls breast development. Some degree of gynaeocomastia is also common in adolescent boys. The average age of onset of menstruation is 13 years.

1. Immediately after birth a newborn baby had a pink body but its hands and feet were blue. The pulse rate was 110 beats/min and respiration slow and irregular. There was a grimace to painful stimuli and some flexion of the limbs.

a. What was the Apgar score?
b. Does this signify permanent brain damage?

2. A newborn infant became progressively jaundiced within 24 hours of birth.

a. Name three causes for the jaundice.
b. Name two serious complications of neonatal jaundice.

3. A mother complained that her toddler was always sleepy and had noisy breathing. On examination, his tongue was always protruding, he looked pale, he was generally slow and had an umbilical hernia.

a. What is the most important diagnosis to exclude?
b. List four other typical physical signs.
c. What test would you request?

4. A 3-year-old became rapidly unwell and developed severe stridor. When his throat was examined, he suddenly became cyanosed.

a. What is the probable diagnosis?
b. What is the causal organism?
c. What treatment is required?

Answers overleaf

1. *a*. Six
b. No, but if the score is still low after 5 min this would be more likely.

2. *a*. (i) Sepsis
(ii) Haemolytic disease of the newborn
(iii) Galactosaemia
b. (i) Deafness
(ii) Kernicterus

3. *a*. Hypothyroidism
b. (i) Puffy eyes
(ii) Sparse hair
(iii) Infantile proportions
(iv) Prolonged tendon reflex relaxation time
c. Serum thyroxine and thyroid stimulating hormone levels

4. *a*. Acute epiglottitis
b. *Haemophilus influenzae*
c. Establishment of an airway (tracheostomy may be required), antibiotics and fluids intravenously

Arrange the following associations into their correct pairs:

1. *A*. Erythema toxicum
B. Neonatal jaundice
C. Cyanosis
D. Anaemia
E. Single umbilical artery

a. Deafness
b. Congenital abnormality of gastrointestinal tract
c. Cephalhaematoma
d. Normal neonatal finding
e. Hypoglycaemia

2. *A*. 'Frog' position
B. Palpable kidneys
C. Single palmar crease
D. Hairy patch on back
E. Hypocalcaemia

a. Down's syndrome
b. Spina bifida occulta
c. Normal neonatal finding
d. Pre-term infant
e. 'Jittery' baby

3. *A*. Macroglossia
B. Webbed neck
C. Bossing of the skull
D. 'Cracked pot' skull percussion note
E. Sunken fontanelle

a. Thalassaemia
b. Dehydration
c. Hypothyroidism
d. Turner's syndrome
e. Raised intracranial pressure

4. *A*. Systolic thrill at lower left sternal edge
B. Continuous murmur
C. Widely split pulmonary second sound
D. Inspiratory splitting of the pulmonary second sound
E. Midsystolic murmur in the 2nd right interspace

a. Aortic stenosis
b. Ventricular septal defect
c. Normal infant
d. Patent ductus arteriosus
e. Atrial septal defect

5. *A*. Mouth ulceration
B. Discoloured teeth
C. Koplik's spots
D. Bright orange tonsils
E. Stridor

a. Tangier disease
b. Hypocalcaemia
c. Leukaemia
d. Tetracycline administration
e. Measles

Answers overleaf

1. *A......d*
B......a
C......e
D......c
E......b

2. *A......d*
B......c
C......a
D......b
E......e

3. *A......c*
B......d
C......a
D......e
E......b

4. *A......b*
B......d
C......e
D......c
E......a

5. *A......c*
B......d
C......e
D......a
E......b